Yang Chengfu

The Essence and Applications of Taijiquan

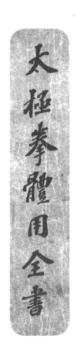

Yang Chengfu

The Essence and Applications of Taijiquan

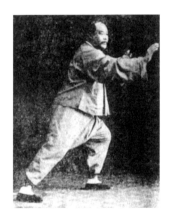

Translated by

Louis Swaim

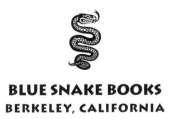

BLUE SNAKE BOOKS
BERKELEY, CALIFORNIA

Published by Blue Snake Books, an imprint of North Atlantic Books
Huichin, unceded Ohlone land
aka Berkeley, California

Cover design by Paula Morrison
Book design by Jan Camp
Printed in Canada

The Essence and Applications of Taijiquan is sponsored and published by North Atlantic Books, an educational nonprofit based in the unceded Ohlone land Huichin (aka Berkeley, CA) that collaborates with partners to develop cross-cultural perspectives; nurture holistic views of art, science, the humanities, and healing; and seed personal and global transformation by publishing work on the relationship of body, spirit, and nature.

North Atlantic Books' publications are distributed to the US trade and internationally by Penguin Random House Publishers Services. For further information, visit our website at www.northatlanticbooks.com

Library of Congress Cataloging-in-Publication Data
Yang, Chengfu, 1883–1936.
 [Taijiquan tiyong quanshu. English]
 The essence and applications of taijiquan / by Yang Chengfu ; translated by Louis Swaim.
    p. cm.
 Summary: "A traditional manual on the Chinese martial art of taijiquan, based on the demonstration narrative of the eminent master, Yang Chengfu. Presents the complete Yang family form, along with interesting application scenarios"—Provided by publisher.
 Includes bibliographical references.
 ISBN 1-55643-545-2 (pbk.)
 ISBN-13: 978-1-55643-545-4
 1. Tai chi. I. Title.
 GV504.Y32 2005
 613.7'148—dc22   2004027497

10 11 12 13 MQ 24 23 22 21

North Atlantic Books is committed to the protection of our environment. We print on recycled paper whenever possible and partner with printers who strive to use environmentally responsible practices.

This book is dedicated
to the memory of my father,
John Wesley Swaim.

Acknowledgments

My work on this book translation began some years ago, and because of various commitments, I was only able to pursue it in spare moments over time. During that time, I benefited from many discussions with friends. Some of the people who have either encouraged me—or challenged me to clarify and re-think my approach to translating—include Jerry Karin, Audi Peal, Jeff Crosland, and a host of contributors to online discussions. Barbara Davis, Douglas Wile, and Jeff Crosland each read late drafts of the manuscript, and generously offered detailed suggestions for its improvement. Kathy Glass copyedited the manuscript with grace and efficiency. I, of course, am responsible for any remaining oversights or errors of interpretation.

Jess O'Brien often encouraged me, and gently nudged me to complete the project, always knowing exactly what to say, and what not to say. The staff and associates of North Atlantic Books, including Jan Camp, Paula Morrison, and Yvonne Cardenas worked smoothly and professionally to carry the book through to production.

I wish to thank my mom and my sisters for the support that only family can give. My daughter Emma, with her thirst for knowledge, love of literature, and zest for life, has been a constant inspiration.

Table of Contents

Translator's Introduction ix

    Conventions. xvi

    Notes. xvi

Zheng Manqing's Foreword 1

    Notes. 3

Yang Chengfu's Preface 7

Yang Chengfu's Introduction 10

    Notes. 13

Yang Shouzhong's Preface 19

Taijiquan Form Sections 21

Push Hands and *Dalu* Sections 103

    Illustrated Explanation of the *Dalu* Forms. 109

Appendix: Taijiquan Classics 113

    I. The Taijiquan Treatise 113

    II. Song of the Thirteen Postures 115

    III. The Mental Elucidation of the Thirteen Postures. 116

    IV. The Taijiquan Classic 117

    V. The Song of Pushing Hands .119

Bibliography 121

Translator's Introduction

The publication in 1934 of Yang Chengfu's book, *Essence and Applications of Taijiquan (Taijiquan tiyong quanshu)*, marked a milestone in the modern evolution of the art of taijiquan. It is the written culmination of Yang's teachings on the art. Yet, as popular as taijiquan has grown to be, few taijiquan enthusiasts in the West know anything about the contents of this seminal book. There are a number of likely reasons that this source has been overlooked for so long. For one, the book is difficult to translate, since it is written in a style that is distilled and compact — a presentation that differs from speech or vernacular writing, and that includes frequent classical or literary turns of phrase that remain obscure unless the reader is familiar with, or can discover, the sources from whence they came. In addition, there are numerous problems in the features and organization of the text that cause difficulties of interpretation. Finally, there are questions about the authorship of the book that need clarification. In my approach to this book translation, I have tried to address each of these issues in a way that I hope will help the modern taijiquan enthusiast to get a grasp of Yang's valuable insights.

Early published manuals on taijiquan from the 1920s and 1930s should be understood within a greater context of a gradual evolution from oral tradition and highly codified written texts that were privately transmitted, to more explicit notation of detailed body mechanics that were publicly transmitted. The kind of detailed kinesiological description witnessed in modern manuals (written in the late 1950s and early 1960s), such as those by Fu Zhongwen or Gu Liuxin, were strongly influenced by advances in formalized physical education instruction.[1] The earliest written taiji documents, such as what we now call "the classics," are probably best understood as supplementary adjuncts to personal, oral instruction. These fit into a common mold with historical Chinese military training manuals, archery manuals, and the like.[2] The earliest taiji texts functioned less as explicit descriptions of movement than as distillations of experiential principles. They might be viewed as a sort of "prompt book" for advanced students and masters.

An analog in Chinese literary tradition is a body of literature known as *huaben* (talk book) stories. *Huaben* literature most likely came out of a tradition of teahouse storytellers. The storytelling art was passed down from master to student, or within a family tradition. Slowly, a written tradition developed that recorded the stories in a bare bones and formulaic presentation, whose sole purpose was to preserve the outlines of the stories and to serve as a memory prompt. Later, these prompt books were built upon and fleshed out into more narrative form by literary-minded writers for publication. Thus what had been accessible to the public only through teahouse storytellers now became available to a reading public as a sort of proto-novel.

If the classical texts of taijiquan represent subjective experience expressed through the insightful records of early masters, the later manuals represent a more objective, distanced, and analytical approach to the physical movements. Yang Chengfu's *Taijiquan tiyong quanshu* occupies a transitional position somewhere between the earlier "experiential" texts and the later physical education-oriented manuals. As such, it provides a rare glimpse into the direct, hands-on teaching of the art by Yang Chengfu by means of what is best termed "demonstration narrative." That is, it is a record of Yang going through the form, section by section, demonstrating the functional aspects of the art while simultaneously explaining the applications. Each section consists of a photo of Yang Chengfu in the sequenced ending posture, accompanied by a narrative describing a suggested application scenario. In most cases, the scenario begins with words such as, "Suppose the opponent strikes at me with his left hand," then proceeds with the suggested application. Each posture is treated as a separate scenario. A perfunctory linkage from one section to the next is effected with introductory phrases such as "From the previous posture, suppose an opponent comes from behind me. . . ." In some cases, but not all, the linkages give logical insight into the transitional moves from posture to posture. The perspective is clearly that of Yang Chengfu, perhaps demonstrating with one of his students responding to cues and striking or feinting at Yang accordingly. Once the reader understands this context of "demonstration narrative," the teachings of Yang Chengfu will come across with an immediacy and liveliness unavailable before.

The suggested scenarios should by no means be construed as the exclusive or definitive applications for their given forms. In fact, Yang's narrative occasionally suggests alternate scenarios of response, depending upon the potentially changing circumstances of the attack. One of the values of the text is the emphasis it places upon maintaining postural alignment and equilibrium, while seeking strategies to unbalance and overcome the opponent. Rather than providing an inventory of martial techniques, the suggested scenarios only help to illustrate how the advanced taijiquan practitioner can develop these deeper strategies.

If the form narratives in fact represent the direct teachings of Yang Chengfu, one might ask how it is they came to be recorded in book form. It has long been speculated that the book was actually ghostwritten by Zheng Manqing (Cheng Man-ch'ing). Yang Chengfu's second son, Yang Zhenji, made it quite clear when he stated, "*Taijiquan tiyong quanshu* was written by my father's disciple, Zheng Manqing, according to my father's performance narratives and requirements. This is factual."[3] Yang Zhenji thus makes it clear that the basis of the book was his father's "performance narratives" (*yanshu* 演述). However, one must dig a little deeper to clarify Zheng's role in writing the book. To this end, I have compared the form section texts of *Taijiquan tiyong quanshu* with an earlier book published in 1931 under Yang Chengfu's name, *Taijiquan shiyongfa* (Application Methods of Taijiquan). That book is known to have been compiled and edited by another of Yang's students, Dong Yingjie (Tung Ying-chieh).[4] The earlier version was likely an assemblage of observations and notes collected over time from Yang Chengfu's teaching sessions. These "class notes" were then distilled into Dong's terse, semi-classical style of writing.

One immediate difference between the texts is that the earlier *Shiyongfa* sections are unpunctuated, while the form sections for *Taijiquan tiyong quanshu* have punctuation. Traditional Chinese books were not punctuated, and it was the reader's job to parse the sentences, determine which clauses were subordinate, and to match up subjects and predicates. Dong Yingjie was a classically trained scholar and evidently did not feel compelled to use punctuation in his writing. However, among the many changes in society and education during China's encounter with modernity, there came the introduction in the early twentieth century of Western-style punctuation (*biaodian* 標點). Increasingly, modern readers who were not trained in reading classical Chinese writings relied upon punctuation for their comprehension. The addition of punctuation in Yang's later book was evidently an editorial decision on Zheng Manqing's part. Zheng was classically trained, but he must have felt the need to make the book more accessible to modern readers.

In many cases, the added punctuation is the *only* difference between the earlier and later form section texts. In other cases, some rough or ambiguous wording has been smoothed or reworked. Finally, in a number of cases, there are identifiable qualitative changes and additions. These include cases where there are added allusions to literary or philosophical texts that we know Zheng was versed in. Most educated Chinese at the time would have had at least passing familiarity with Zheng's allusions to such texts as the *Zhuangzi*, the *Daodejing*, the *Daxue* or "Greater Learning," and the *Xici*, sometimes called the "Great Commentary" or "Appended

TRANSLATOR'S INTRODUCTION

Phrases" section from the *Book of Changes*. Chinese writers typically did not attribute such quotations. They were simply run into the writer's text with the expectation that the reader would recognize them and know their significance. I have done my best to identify the allusions for the reader. Other changes evidently added by Zheng are what might be termed "envoi" statements frequently used to close the individual sections. These often appear as little formulaic remarks such as, "There is no one who will not fall down" as a result of the given technique, or "This will ensure success." Some of the envoi statements are more expansive than others, and some of them survive in Zheng Manqing's own later book, *Zhengzi taijiquan shisan pian* (Master Zheng's Thirteen Chapters on Taijiquan).

The comparison of the 1934 book, *Taijiquan tiyong quanshu* with the 1931 book, *Taijiquan shiyongfa,* clearly indicates that Zheng Manqing's role was to edit and polish the earlier version. A statement in Yang Chengfu's "Introduction" supports this: "This book is based on the previous books, revised and corrected, to remain as a standard model." The underlying demonstration narrative is substantially the same in both books, and its structure strongly suggests that it was a direct record of Yang Chengfu's own teachings.

While there appears to be a strong case accounting for the development of the main form description section of the book, it is less clear how the sections on push hands and *dalu* developed, and to what degree they reflect Yang Chengfu's direct narratives. These sections do seem to be consistent with the "demonstration narrative" model, but the descriptions in *Taijiquan tiyong quanshu* differ rather substantially from those in the earlier book. The earlier book, *Taijiquan shiyongfa,* also included a separate applications *(shiyongfa)* section, with descriptions of martial applications for some of the major sequences of the solo form. These descriptions were accompanied by photos of Yang Chengfu demonstrating the applications with a partner.[5] In addition, the earlier book had sections on a staff

xiii

or spear form, along with several early texts and commentaries not included in *Taijiquan tiyong quanshu*. It may be that some of these materials were to have been incorporated into the proposed second volume on sword and spear methods mentioned in Zheng's foreword and Yang's introduction, but Yang Chengfu died before that volume materialized.

More problematic with regard to authorship are the "Preface" and "Introduction" presented under Yang Chengfu's name. The "Preface" has Yang Chengfu recounting first-hand conversations with his grandfather, Yang Luchan. This is an impossibility, given the fact that Yang Chengfu was born in 1883, eleven years after the date recorded as the year Yang Luchan died: 1872.[6] One could speculate that Zheng wrote the "Preface" and "Introduction" based upon second-hand accounts of Yang family anecdotes. The anecdotes may have been true, save for the awkward anachronism of Yang being in his grandfather's presence. But even apart from this sticky situation, a good deal of the discourse in the alleged conversation seems a better fit with the social and political background of Zheng Manqing than that of Yang Luchan's generation.

A few remarks are in order with regard to the title of the book. The literal translation of the title, *Taijiquan tiyong quanshu* 太極拳體用全書, is *The Complete Book of the Essence and Applications of Taijiquan*. The "complete book" would probably have more accurately applied to the proposed two-volume set, of which only the first book was ever published. The important term in the title is *tiyong* 體用. The term *tiyong* has a long history as a philosophical concept. Its earliest appearance was in a commentary to Laozi's *Daodejing* by Wang Bi (226–249 CE). As a philosophical formulation it has had a varied career, surviving into the late imperial period. It can be variously translated as "theory and application," "structure and function," "essence and practical use," and the like. In early modern China, with the increasingly intrusive presence of Western nations, the *tiyong* formula found new significance as a political slogan during what was called the "self-strengthening" movement — "Chinese learning should remain the essence, but Western learning should be used for practical development." This was a potent formula for preserving cultural identity while appropriating modern military, institutional, and engineering advances needed for national survival.

In taijiquan, the *ti* generally refers to form practice, and the *yong* to practical applications. However, Zheng Manqing may have deliberately used the *tiyong* term because of its resonance with the earlier philosophical meaning as well as its political overtone. After all, here was a method for self-strengthening that affirmed the very best of Chinese cultural essence.[7] Zheng used the *tiyong* term in the title of a poem he wrote, "Tiyong Ge" (Song of Essence and Application), as did Li Yiyu (1832–1892) at an earlier time, "Taijiquan Tiyong Ge" (Song of the Essence and Application of Taijiquan).[8] Early texts among those called the "Yang Family Forty Chapters" include references to the *tiyong* formula, including a brief text titled "Taiji Tiyong Jie" (Explanation of the Essence and Applications of Taiji), and one titled "Taiji Wen Wu Jie" (Explanation of the Civil and Martial in Taiji).[9] The latter correlates the civil (*wen* 文) with essence (*ti* 體), and martial (*wu* 武) with application (*yong* 用). So taijiquan had from an early time incorporated the concept into its theory.

In doing this book translation, my goal has been to bring the teachings of Yang Chengfu to light for modern taijiquan enthusiasts. I have used a comparative approach to try to identify and reveal the direct demonstration narrative as recorded and filtered through his students. I've added commentary where I think it may add interest, ferreting out allusions, cracking the occasional tough nut, and pointing to probable additions from Zheng Manqing's pen. For the sake of historical documentation of the traditional Yang family form, I have made occasional reference to the "received form" as taught by Fu Zhongwen, Yang Zhenji, and Yang Zhenduo, where doing so may clarify some ambiguity or lacunae in the form descriptions as presented. I have also included a few comparative references from the earlier form manual of Xu Yusheng, *Taijiquan shi tujie* (Taijiquan Forms Illustrated), where it sheds light on taiji terminology.

I hope that this book will be a useful study tool for fellow practitioners, as well as a point of departure for future comparative studies of early taijiquan writings. Even more, I hope that the demonstation narratives revealed here will enable taiji enthusiasts to feel closer to the source.

Conventions

I use the Chinese *pinyin* system of romanization for Chinese words, except in some translation excerpts or book titles where an older system was employed. For some technical vocabulary, I use the Chinese term rather than translate each occurrence. For example, I employ the term *kua* throughout the book, which in taijiquan usage refers to the thighs, hips, or hip joints, but is more inclusive than any one of these terms in English. I have avoided using the English term "posture" for the named movements depicted in the photos in this book, preferring the word "form." Posture implies something static, but the sequenced configurations of taijiquan express a dynamic quality that is not well-served by "posture." As I employ the word, "form" can refer to an individual movement configuration, such as "White Crane Displays Wings," or to the entire set of movements from beginning to end: the taijiquan form.

Notes

1. Gu Liuxin (1908–1990) was an innovator in applying modern analytical research methodology to the study of taijiquan history and theory. He played an important role as an acquisitions editor for *Renmin Tiyu Chubanshe* (People's Physical Education Publishing), facilitating the publication of modern manuals for all of the major modern taijiquan styles, including Fu Zhongwen's Yang style manual. For a useful account of the modern development and formalization of physical education (*tiyu* 體育), see Susan Brownell, *Training the Body for China: Sports in*

the Moral Order of the People's Republic (Chicago: University of Chicago Press, 1995).

2. See the excellent study by Stephen Selby, *Chinese Archery* (Hong Kong: Hong Kong University Press, 2000).

3. Yang Zhenji, *Yang Chengfu shi taijiquan,* p. 250.

4. See T.Y. Pang, *On Tai Chi Chuan,* pp. 240–242.

5. See Douglas Wile, *T'ai-chi Touchstones,* for these application photos.

6. See Wile, *T'ai-chi Touchstones,* p. iv, et passim, for additional assessments of the problems in Yang's "Preface."

7. For insightful analysis into taijiquan's public emergence in the self-strengthening context, see Douglas Wile, *Lost T'ai-chi Classics from the Late Ch'ing Dynasty,* pp. 22–30.

8. Zheng's poem is translated in Benjamin Lo, *Cheng Tzu's Thirteen Treatises on T'ai Chi Ch'uan,* pp. 217–218. Li Yiyu's poem is translated in Wile, *Lost T'ai-chi Classics,* pp. 50–51, 130.

9. Wile, *Lost T'ai-chi Classics,* pp. 70–71, 138–139.

鍛鍊身心

澄甫太極專家體用全書

蔣中正題

"Temper and train body and mind."
— Jiang Zhongzheng (Chiang Kai-shek)

國術精華

楊澄甫先生著

太極拳體用全書

吳鐵城

"Essence of our national arts"
—Wu Tiecheng

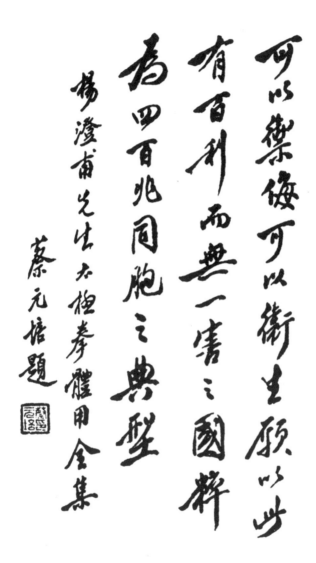

可以禦侮可以衛生願以此
有百利而無一害之國粹
為四百兆同胞之典型
楊澄甫先生太極拳體用全集
蔡元培題

"Averting insults and protecting health, this national treasure has
a hundred benefits for willing students, and will serve as a standard
for four hundred million countrymen."
—Cai Yuanpei

後學楷式

張厲生題

"A model form for students"
—Zhang Lisheng

厲剛于柔

張乃燕題

"Storing the hard in the soft"
— Zhang Naiyan

澄甫先生太極體用全書

龍騰虎臥

吳思豫題

"The dragon leaps; the tiger sleeps."
—Wu Siyu

自強不息

張人傑題

"Strengthen yourselves without cease."
—Zhang Renjie

民族精神

龐炳勳

"Vital spirt of our people"
—Pang Bingxun

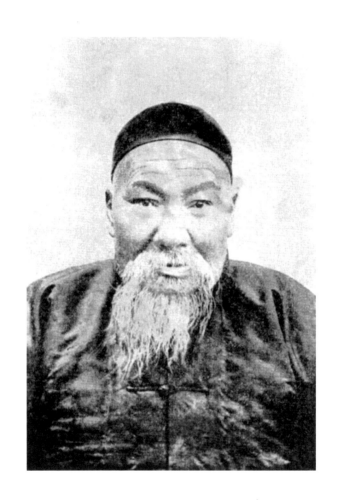

Yang Jianhou

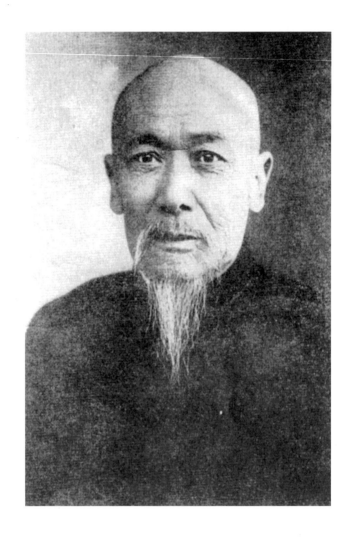

Yang Shaohou

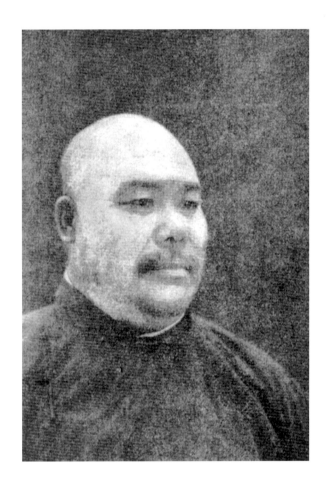

Author, Yang Chengfu

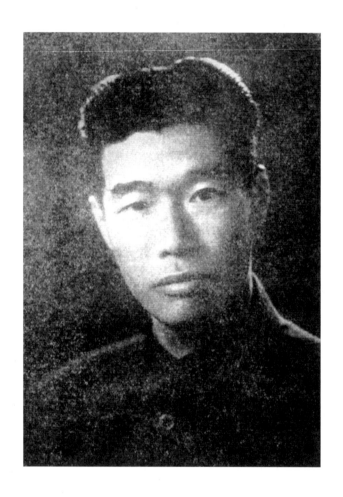

Yang Shouzhong

Zheng Manqing's Foreword

In the natural realm, only by the hardest can one prevail over the softest, and yet it is only by the softest that one can prevail over the hardest. The *Book of Changes* says, "Hard and soft stroke each other, the eight trigrams stimulate each other."[1] The *Book of Documents* says, "The reserved and retiring are subdued with strength, those of lofty intelligence are subdued with gentleness."[2] The *Book of Songs* says, "Neither devour the soft nor reject the hard."[3] If it is so that all of these follow the same principles in the applications of hard and soft, how is it that Laozi alone said, "In the natural realm, the softest things ride roughshod over the firmest"?[4] And, "The soft and weak win over the hard and strong"?[5] I was highly skeptical about this.

At the end of the Song Dynasty the sage Zhang Sanfeng created the technique of taiji soft fist, with what is called "having *qi*, then there is no strength; not having *qi*, then there is pure hardness."[6] Is this not strange? I felt that this concept seemed even more at odds with Laozi's theory in particular, and asked, "Why is this so?" I certainly already knew of the softness that comes through not using strength, but had not heard that there was such a thing as not using *qi*. If one doesn't use *qi*, how indeed can one have strength, and then attain pure hardness?

In 1923, I assumed a teaching position at Beijing Fine Arts Academy. A colleague, Liu Yongchen, was good at this art of taijiquan. Because I was emaciated and weak, he urged me to study. Barely a month passed before I had to quit because of important commitments, so I was not able to catch on to the art.

In the spring of 1930, because of overwork while establishing the China Academy of Literature and Arts, I had reached the point of coughing up blood, so I resumed study and practice of taijiquan with my colleagues Xiao Zhongbo and Ye Dami. In less than a month, my illness swiftly subsided, and my constitution became stronger daily. From that point on, I practiced day and night with steady efforts. Within two years, when I matched up with men ten times my strength, I could beat several of them! I was beginning to believe that softness was sufficient to defeat hardness, but still didn't understand the subtlety of not using *qi*.

In the first lunar month of 1932, I met Master Yang Chengfu at Mr. Pu Qiuzhen's house. After the old gentleman had introduced me, I humbly presented myself at Master Yang's door, and received his teachings, including his oral instructions of the inner work. I began to understand the meaning of not using *qi!* By not using *qi,* I follow the flow, while the other goes against the flow. One has only to follow, then softly yield. The way that softness subdues hardness is gradual, while the way hardness subdues softness is abrupt. Abruptness is easy to detect, and so it is easily defeated. It is more difficult to sense gradualness, so it often prevails. This notion of not using *qi* is the extreme of softness. Only the extreme of softness can produce extreme hardness.

When I reached this, I came to understand. It was, after all, consistent with the treatises of the sage (Zhang Sanfeng) and Laozi, and with the teachings of the *Book of Changes* about the resonant exchange of hard and soft.

I was still afraid that those hearing my words would share the feelings of doubt that I once had, when I sought for explanations and proof. So my fellow student Kuang Keming and I went together to Master Yang Chengfu and said, "The methods of the former masters were passed on from generation to generation, all relying on direct oral instruction. There were no specialized manuals. In order to keep the transmission within the family they held the methods close. How would it be to write the methods down in a book so as to ensure the transmission to later generations?" Master Yang agreed that this was a good idea.

Accordingly, here are the ingenious methods of the form and its functions, with complete explanation of its key points through Master Yang's photos and sequence narratives, including detailed analysis. In time there will be a companion volume of sword and spear methods, in which Master Yang exhibits the marvelous skill of "whirling his ax with a noise like the wind" *(yun jin cheng feng).*[7]

In compiling the narrative and producing the book, these are divided into a two-volume work. For all those who want to maintain their health and develop their character, there will be a volume for each hand, making it as clear as one's own palm. This will not only dispel doubts, but can be a technique for strengthening oneself and the nation. It is all to be found in here!

— 1933, Dragon Boat Festival (fifth of the fifth lunar month) Respectfully submitted by Zheng Yue of Yong Jia

Notes

1. The quotation is actually from the *Xici* commentary to the *Book of Changes.* See Richard John Lynn, trans., *The Classic of Changes: A New Translation of the I Ching* (New York: Columbia University Press, 1994), p. 48.

2. My translation, based on: James Legge, trans., *The Chinese Classics,* Vol. III, *The Shoo King,* V:IV:17 p. 333.

3. Zheng's quote as printed, which reorders some of the wording, comes from a stanza of the poem "Zheng Min," which Legge translates,
"The people have a saying: —
'The soft is devoured,
And the hard is ejected from the mouth.'
But Chung Shan-foo
Does not devour the soft,
Nor eject the powerful.

He does not insult the poor or the widow;

He does not fear the strong or the oppressive."

—Legge, trans., *The Chinese Classics,* Vol. IV, *The She King,* III:3:6 pp. 543–544.

4. *Daodejing,* chapter 43.

5. *Daodejing,* chapter 36.

6. The quotation is from the last few lines of Wu Yuxiang's "Mental Elucidation of the Thirteen Postures." Zheng's partial quote is a bit misleading, as the phrases "having *qi*" (*you qi* 有氣) and "not having *qi*" (*wu qi zhe* 無氣者) seem here to stand on their own, while in fact in the original document they are syntactically linked to antecedent phrases, so that they have to do with where the taijiquan practitioner places his or her intent (*yi* 意): "Throughout the whole body, the intent *(yi)* is on the spirit of vitality (*jingshen* 精神), not on the *qi* (*bu zai qi* 不在氣). If it is on the *qi*, then there will be stagnation (*zai qi, ze zhi* 在氣則滯)." Therefore the phrases in question read: "One who has it on the *qi* (*you qi zhe* 有氣者) will have no strength. One who does not have it on the *qi* (*wu qi zhe* 無氣者) will attain pure hardness." Zheng's entire discussion of the notion of "not having *qi,*" and "not using *qi*" is evidently an example of rhetorical exaggeration to emphasize the idea of not taking the initiative in using force against an opponent. The phrase "not using *qi*" (*wu yong qi* 無用氣), in fact, does not occur in any traditional taijiquan documents so far as I can ascertain.

7. The phrase *yun jin cheng feng* (運斤成風) is a *chengyu,* or proverbial phrase, that describes great adeptness. It is based on a marvelous story in the *Zhuangzi,* in which Zhuangzi pays tribute to his late friend and worthy debate adversary, Huizi, by relating a story of two friends. Watson translates the story:

"There was once a plasterer who, if he got a speck of mud on the tip of his nose no thicker than a fly's wing, would get his friend Carpenter Shih to slice it off for him. Carpenter Shih, whirling his hatchet with a noise like the wind [*yun jin cheng feng* 運斤成風],

would accept the assignment and proceed to slice, removing every bit of mud without injury to the nose, while the plasterer just stood there completely unperturbed. Lord Yuan of Sung, hearing of this feat, summoned Carpenter Shih and said, 'Could you try performing it for me?' But Carpenter Shih replied, 'It's true that I was once able to slice like that—but the material I worked on has been dead these many years.' Since you died, Master Hui, I have no material to work on. There's no one I can talk to any more." —Burton Watson, trans., *The Complete Works of Chuang Tzu* (New York: Columbia University Press, 1968), p. 269.

Yang Chengfu's Preface

When I was young I would see my late grandfather, Mr. Yang Luchan, leading my uncles, relatives, and followers in their earnest daily taijiquan training. Some in solo form training, some in partner practice, they practiced day and night without cease. Intellectually, I harbored doubts, considering it like the method of only engaging one enemy, which Xiang Ji scorned learning.[1] For me, I would one day undertake the study of engaging ten thousand enemies.

When I had grown a bit older, my late uncle, Banhou, directed me to study with him. Later, no longer able to conceal my doubts, I told him my honest opinion. My late father, Jianhou, angrily denounced my thinking, saying, "Oh, what kind of talk is that? Your grandfather handed this art down as our family's legacy. Now you want to abandon our vocation *(zhui jiqiu)!*"[2] Grandfather quickly stopped him, saying, "This is not something you can force on a child." He soothed me with his hand and said,

> Sit down and let me tell you. This art that I practice and teach to others is not for taking on enemies, but for protecting one's body. It is not for saving the world, but for helping the nation. The gentlemen *(junzi)* of today know only that our nation's troubles come from poverty; they still do not understand that our nation's sickness lies in its weakness. Therefore, those formulating our national policies vie for plans to save us from poverty, but I have yet to hear a plan to rouse the failing or raise up the weakened. Yet this country is riddled with disease. Who can respond by taking up this great responsibility? This longstanding weakness, then, is this poverty;

poverty in fact originates in weakness. Looking at the growing strength in the various nations, there are none that do not take strengthening their people as the first step. Without even mentioning the grandeur and distinction of Europe and America, there is also the island nation of the dwarf Japanese, who while surely short in physique are yet strong and unyielding.[3] When matched face-to-face with the gaunt and emaciated men of our nation, in deciding victory or defeat, is there any need for divination on what the outcome would be? If so, then the proper path for saving the nation is certainly to recognize the urgency of saving ourselves from weakness. To neglect this, one may as well have no plan, for it is like treating only the surface *(yi yi mo)*.[4]

Since I was young, I have taken on saving the weak as my responsibility. I have often seen marketplace martial artists *(mai jie zhe)* with vitality and physique by no means inferior to so-called strongmen *(dalishi)*, or proponents of *bushido*.[5] I was thrilled, and inquired into their arts, but they were secretive and unobliging.

Now I understand that China herself has self-strengthening arts, yet on the whole we have come to this weakened condition. Is this without a reason?

Later, I heard of the boxing reputation of the Chen family in Henan's Chenjiagou, so I made the long trek there to study with Master Chen Changxing. Although I did not meet with refusal at the gate, quite some time passed before I was permitted to glimpse the advanced stages of the art *(tang'ao)*.[6] With patience, I endured more than ten years. The master was moved by my sincerity, and began, when the moon was bright and everyone was quiet, to reveal the true inside secrets.

When I had completed my studies, I came to the capital, and made a vow to fulfil my aspiration to teach people openly. Before long, I began to see that among my students, the emaciated and weak began to fill out and the sick became healthy. I was greatly pleased. It occurred to me that what one person can teach has a limit, and may be likened to the simple old man who moved the mountain *(yu gong yishan)*.[7] Furthermore, for those of my father's generation and their various followers, if their will was on being of some use in the world, wouldn't they have chosen not to learn this technique for helping the world if they had looked down upon it?

Thereupon, I began suddenly to understand my grandfather's great diligence at this art. Moreover, as for continuing the family heritage, in fact I felt it was imperative, so I gladly requested instruction.

My late grandfather further said,

> Taijiquan was created by Zhang Sanfeng of the late Song Dynasty, and was transmitted through the elders Wang Zongyue, Chen Zhoutong, Zhang Songxi, and Jiang Fa, each succeeding the other without interruption. Chen Changxin was Mr. Jiang Fa's only disciple. Their art was based on what is natural, and took form in a way never far from *Taiji* (great polarity). It comprised thirteen fundamental forms, but the moving applications are inexhaustible. The movement is of the body, and reaches the spiritual. Therefore, unless one accomplishes long training, it will be difficult to obtain the subtle knowledge. I am not lacking in students, yet it is difficult to say even if Banhou is among those who have obtained the consummate skill *(lu huo chun qing)*.[8] Still, when discussing the strengthening of one's self *(qiang shen)*, one day yields one day's benefits; one year yields one year's results. Once a child understands this, he will be able to carry out my wish.

I respectfully recount this, for I dare not forget it. From that point on, I worked with unrelenting effort through twenty hot summers.[9] Now my grandfather, uncle, and father have all passed on from this life.

I thus began to accept students in Beijing, but soon felt cramped and confined, so that results were somewhat limited. So I moved to the Fujian/Zhejiang region. Later I asked my student, Chen Weiming, to publish a book based on my oral instructions. Now more than ten years have passed, and taijiquan's influence has spread to the north and south of the Yellow River, and to the east and west of the Yangzi, and even to the reaches of Guangdong. The numbers of students have increased greatly. Thinking now about Mr. Chen Weiming's book, it only explains the process of training the solo form. Moreover, in reviewing my form postures of ten years ago, they are not as good as today's. From this one can see the limitless quality of this art.

Today, at the request of my students, I am following through by compiling the complete methodology of form and function into a complete volume, including the fundamental training method, plus *tuishou* and *dalu,* and I've added the most recent photographs. I am committing this to print in order to make it available to the public. A second volume on sword, staff, spear, and saber is planned for future publication. I would not dare use my art for self-promotion. I only wish to convey the will of my forebears to rouse the people to help the world.

—Yang Chengfu (Zhaoqing), Guangping, spring of 1933

Yang Chengfu's Introduction

The essential idea in compiling this book is to pay attention to both the form and the function.[10] Every day, the numbers of people learning taijiquan increase. Without an understanding of the methods of form and function, very few will obtain any benefit to mind or body. Therefore, it is not that I value this art as a sentimental attachment; rather I wish that worthy individuals with the highest aspiration will use it for the purpose of self-strengthening. Let us encourage each other as fellow countrymen.

Taijiquan is based on the *taiji* and *bagua* of the *Book of Changes,* and the ideas of *li* (principles), *qi* (energy), and *xiang* (image) help to give shape to these concepts.[11] Confucius said of the *Changes,* "Modelled on heaven and earth's transformations, it never goes beyond them."[12] How does this come out of *li, qi,* and *xiang?* It is only that *li, qi,* and *xiang* are the unfinished beginnings of taijiquan. When one is able to realize all three, then the form and function are integrated. Thus, *xiang* takes its model from the *taiji* and the *bagua. Qi* does not depart from *yin* and *yang,* hard and soft. *Li* orders what is changeless in change so that one may thoroughly know transformation. Students must especially begin by seeking the *xiang* in order to nurture the *qi.* Given time, they will come to understand the *li* spontaneously.

The most important principle in taijiquan is the value placed on the regularity of movement and stillness. Therefore when practicing, the height of one's stance, the swiftness or slowness with which one extends one's hand, the lightness or heaviness of movement, the stretching and contracting of one's advances and retreats, the broadness or fineness of one's breathing, the attention from left to right or from up to down, the alignment of waist, head-top, back, and abdomen—one must know that for each of these there is a consistent measure. You cannot be suddenly high and suddenly low, suddenly swift and suddenly slow, suddenly light and suddenly heavy, suddenly extending and suddenly contracting, suddenly broad and suddenly fine, suddenly turning left and right, or leaning to and fro without evenness. Only when the height of the stance and the velocity of our hands can obtain this consistent measure can one shed the constraints of fixed rules.

Generally speaking, there are thirteen important points in taijiquan. These are: Sink the shoulders and drop the elbows; contain the chest and pull up the back; the *qi* sinks to the *dantian;* an intangible energy lifts the crown of the head; loosen the waist and *kua;* distinguish empty and full; upper and lower follow one another; use mind intent, not strength; inner and outer are united; intention and *qi* interact; seek stillness in movement; movement and stillness are united; and, proceed evenly from posture to posture. These thirteen points must be attended to in each and every movement. One cannot neglect the concept of these thirteen points within any of the postures. I hope that students will be cautiously attentive, and test and verify these in their practice.

The applications in this book are for those who have already become proficient in taijiquan and wish to progress further. Thus, one need not adhere to fixed orientations, and may experiment with all four sides and corners. If there are those who have not trained thoroughly in the form, they should not skip stages and practice applications. I'm afraid they would simply lack a foundation, and the end results would be few.

As for beginners, I hope they will carefully go over the illustrations of the solo form. With time, as you become refined in all of the basic requirements, the applications will not be difficult to learn.

There is only one school of taijiquan; there are not two ways of learning. One may not make a show of one's cleverness by rashly making additions or deletions. The former worthies developed these methods. If alterations or corrections could be made, the ancestors preceding me would already have put them into effect. Why wait for our generation? I hope that later students will not merely chase after the externals, but will instead pursue what is internal. If you want to attain the highest achievement, have some patience and it will come. The important fine details of the boxing postures cannot be obtained in the appearance of form, but must be sought in the idea that unites the whole. This book is based on the previous books, revised and corrected, to remain as a standard model.

Taijiquan was not created just to engage in quarrels or tests of strength. Perhaps the sage Sanfeng created soft boxing to use in increasing our store of good health *(zizhu daoti)*.[13] People who wish to protect their bodies *(weishen)*, and cultivate their nature *(yang xing)*, to prevent illness and promote longevity, no matter whether they are literati *(sao ren moke)*, whether emaciated and weak, old or young, women or men, all can study this art.[14] Those with perseverance can accomplish results within three years.

If we ask what the use of this art is, it rests in not using strength, and yet not fearing the strong. If someone with great strength comes to attack me, I rely on the greatest pliancy *(zhi rou).*[15] That will be sufficient to prevail, for I just follow his tendency *(shi)* and take it from him.[16] One could indeed say that the core of protecting the body and cultivating our nature is to accord with and protect its weakness.[17] Even if you could possess boldness and strength equal to that of Meng Ben and Xia Yu, this is not something a taijiquan practitioner would choose to emulate.[18]

When beginning study of this boxing form, one must not be too greedy. If each day you only carefully practice one or two postures, then it will be easy to glimpse their inner secrets. Those seeking too much will only get superficial information.

When you have completed practice, don't immediately sit down. You should walk around a bit in order to regulate the *qi* and the blood.

Upon completing practice in the heat of summer, don't use cool water to wash your hands; it could cause a stagnation of fire. When finished with practice in the deep cold of winter, be quick to put on extra clothing to avoid catching cold. Your efforts *(gongfu)* should increase during times of cold and heat. There's a saying, "Train in the dog days of summer and the coldest days of winter." The sun at these times is in a stronger position than in spring and autumn. One must not neglect the times just after arising from bed in the morning and directly before going to bed at night. In this way, your efforts will easily begin to show results.

Taiji sword, spear, saber, lance, and so forth should follow in sequence for publication for fellow enthusiasts.

Notes

1. The reference is to a biography of Xiang Ji, also known as Xiang Yu, in Han historian Sima Qian's *Shiji.* Here is the relevant passage:

    "When Hsiang Yu was a boy he studied the art of writing. Failing to master this, he abandoned it and took up swordsmanship. When he failed at this also, his uncle, Hsiang Liang, grew angry with him, but Hsiang Yu declared, 'Writing is good only for keeping records of people's names. Swordsmanship is useful only for attacking a single enemy and is likewise not worth studying. What I want to learn is the art of attacking ten thousand enemies!'" — Burton Watson, trans., *Records of the Historian: Chapters from the Shih chi of Ssu-ma Ch'ien* (New York: Columbia University Press, 1969), p. 68.

2. "abandon our vocation" — The phrase *jiqiu* 箕裘 is a very arcane way of referring to an inherited family trade, and to the gradual process involved in its transmission. The phrase comes from two sentences in the "Record of Learning" chapter of the *Liji:* "The son of a good founder is sure to learn how to make a fur-robe (*qiu* 裘). The son of a good maker of bows is sure to learn how to make a sieve (*ji* 箕)." Legge, trans., *Li Chi: Book of Rites,* Vol. II (New Hyde Park: University Books, 1967), p. 90.

3. Historically, "dwarf" (*zhuru* 侏儒) was a term of disparagement for the Japanese, which had again gained currency in response to the Japanese occupation of China. While the term is undeniably a slur, it is clear that the intent here is ironic — expressing a grudging admiration for Japan's accomplishments in modernizing.

4. "treating only the surface" — The phrase *"yimo"* (抑末) refers to the tips of the branches, as opposed to the root. A passage in the Analects illustrates the usage: "Ziyou said, 'The disciples and young friends of Zixia are quite all right when it comes to housekeeping, taking care of guests, and standing in attendance, but these are just the tips of the branches. What do you do about the fact that they have no roots?'" — Roger Ames and Henry Rosemont, Jr., trans., *The Analects of Confucius: A Philosophical Translation* (New York: Ballantine, 1998), 19:12, pp. 220–221.

5. "marketplace martial artists" — The term *maijie* (賣解) refers to acrobats and martial artists who perform for fairs and marketplaces. The term *dalishi* (大力士) refers to Western-style strongmen such as Hercules, while *bushido* (武士道 *wushidao* in Chinese) refers to the Japanese warrior ethos. Many Chinese thinkers in the early eighteenth century had an admiring fascination for *bushido*. The important

reformer, Liang Qichao, wrote a popular book in 1904, *Zhongguo zhi wushidao* (Chinese Bushido), which sought to reinvigorate China's indigenous martial ethos. See Hao Chang, *Liang Ch'i-ch'ao and Intellectual Transition in China, 1890–1907* (Cambridge: Harvard University Press, 1971), p. 278.

6. "advanced stages" — Literally, *tang'ao* (堂奧) refers to the southwest interior corner of a home, where a family altar may be kept. By extension, it is the place of honor and respect, or hidden and treasured knowledge.

7. "The Simple Old Man Who Moved a Mountain." This refers to a parable that every Chinese child learns in school, about the importance of perseverance and determination in accomplishing a task. The story first appeared in the *Liezi*, where "Mr. Simple" *(Yu Gong),* at the age of ninety, proposed to his family that they endeavor to move a mountain that was inconveniently in the way. When met with skepticism, he replied,

> "Even when I die, I shall have sons surviving me. My sons will beget me more grandsons, my grandsons in their turn will have sons, and these will have more sons and grandsons. My descendants will go on for ever, but the mountains will get no bigger. Why should there be any difficulty about levelling it?" — A. C. Graham, trans., *The Book of Lieh-tzu: A Classic of Tao* (New York: Columbia University Press, 1990), p. 100.

8. "consummate skill" *(lu huo chun qing* 爐火純青) lit., "the stove fire for concocting the elixir of life begins to give a pure glow." This saying comes out of Daoist tradition.

9. "unrelenting effort" — *(qie er bu she* 鍥而不舍), lit., "carve without giving up," from Xunzi's "Exhortation to Learning." "If you start carving but give up, you cannot cut even a rotting piece of wood in two. Yet if you carve away and never give up, even metal and stone can be engraved." (John Knoblock, trans., *Xunzi: A Translation and Study of the Complete Works, Volume I*, p. 138.)

10. "Form and function" here translate *tiyong* 體用. See my general comments on the historical uses of the term in the Translator's Introduction.

11. This trio of terms, *li* 理, *qi* 氣, and *xiang* 象, is likely inspired by the *Xici* commentary to the *Book of Changes*, but it is not immediately clear what the author's intent is in using them in the context of learning taijiquan. The word *xiang* 象 is most often translated "image," and it should be understood as "a sensory (that is, visual, auditory, tactile, olfactory) presentation of a perceptual, imaginative, or recollected experience." (Hall and Ames, *Anticipating China*, p. 216.) The *Xici* states, "Therefore, as for the images [*xiang* 象], the sages had the means to perceive the mysteries of the world and, drawing comparisons to them with analogous things, made images out of those things that seemed appropriate. In consequence of this, they called these 'images.'" (Richard John Lynn, *The Classic of Changes*, p. 68.) *Qi* 氣 in this context is the basic material force of life, at once matter and energy. The word *li* 理 here refers to the inherent principles of things, or their structural patterns. Roger Ames writes, "One investigates *li* in order to uncover patterns which relate things, and to discover resonances between things that make correlations and categorization possible." (Hall and Ames, *ibid.*, p. 214.) In the taijiquan context, it may be helpful to think of *xiang* as learning through emulation of a teacher's model form. It begins to become meaningful at the immediate level when one can "nurture" one's *qi* (養氣), or energetic sense of the form. Then, in time, one gradually becomes more intimate with the internal principles of the art.

12. This is actually a quote from the *Xici* commentary, and there is not universal agreement on whether these are the words of Confucius. See Rutt, *Zhouyi: The Book of Changes*, p. 411.

13. "increasing our store of good health" — The author's use of these two compound phrases, *zizhu* (資助) and *daoti* (道體), is interesting. The term *zizhu* generally means "to assist," but is often used in the economic sense of "to subsidize," "to fund," or "to supply." The phrase *daoti* is a Daoist term meaning "the essence of the Dao," but as "the body of the Dao," the phrase has an extended meaning as an honorific or polite reference to another's health. In Daoist philosophy, the body is at once individual and collective; one could say that taking care

of the body is taking care of the community. Given the reference to Zhang Sanfeng, the use of the term *daoti* has obvious Daoist overtones, but it takes on an added layer of meaning *vis-à-vis* the background political discourse of self-strengthening, as "body politic."

14. "to protect their bodies" — The term *weishen* (衛身) is not a standard term for self-defense (*ziwei* 自衛), but serves nicely here to denote both martial self-defense and protection of health. For "cultivate their nature" (*yangxing* 養性), see Mengzi, 7:1:2 — "To preserve one's mental constitution, and nourish one's nature, is the way to serve Heaven." Legge, trans., *The Chinese Classics*, Vol. II, *The Works of Mencius*, pp. 448–449. The term for "literati," *sao ren moke* 騷人墨客, derives from the poem "Li Sao," by 4th century BC poet Qu Yuan.

15. "greatest pliancy" — The term *zhi rou* 至柔 (arriving at softness/pliancy, attained softness, the softest) is from the *Daodejing*. It appears in chapter 10 in the sentence, "In concentrating your *qi* and attaining pliancy *(zhirou)*, are you able to become the newborn babe?" See also chapter 43, "In the natural realm, the softest things ride roughshod over the firmest." Chen Weiming used the term *zhirou* for the name of his school in Shanghai.

16. "tendency" — The word *shi* 勢 can be variously translated as "position," "configuration," "power," "force," etc. Here, the meaning is "tendency," as in "directional tendency." For a thorough exploration of the meaning of *shi*, see Francois Jullien, *The Propensity of Things*. See also Roger Ames, *The Art of Rulership*, and Ralph D. Sawyer's synoptic note in his *The Seven Military Classics of Ancient China*, pp. 429–432, n. 37.

17. The phrase "protect its weakness" (*shou qi ruo* 守其弱) could be an oblique reference to a line in chapter 52 of the *Daodejing*, "Safeguarding the pliant is real strength (*shou rou yue qiang* 守柔曰強)." Both *ruo* 弱 (weakness) and *rou* 柔 (softness, pliancy) are used in the *Daodejing*, and are closely associated in meaning.

18. The author uses the combined form, *"Ben-Yu,"* a literary convention referring to Meng Ben and Xia Yu, who were famous warriors from the Warring States period, known for their strength.

Yang Shouzhong's Preface

While he was staying in Guangdong, my father authored this book at the request of his comrades to clearly set forth the essence and applications of taijiquan. Since taijiquan is based upon the *Yijing's taiji* and *bagua*, and its accomplishments draw upon the *li* (principles), *qi* (energy), and *xiang* (image), students must first seek the *xiang* in order to nurture the *qi*. With time, one will come to understand the principles on one's own. Therefore, my father recorded in detail each form and posture to facilitate its study. Perhaps it will help to clarify the essence and identify the applications, in order to arrive at a state of sudden understanding. Students truly must not ignore this!

The first edition was printed in 1934. Then, in all too short a time, my father passed away. Now it is more than ten years later, and China has been through the War of Resistance (1937–45). Many people have since been scattered and lost. I, Shouzhong, am a dull sort, and am hard pressed to carry on the achievements of my forebears. I long for the days of the past, and wipe away the tears of sadness. Now I take these printing plates which still exist, with a plan for a new edition. Having had the pleasure of friendly support, I am able to bring it to publication. The entire book is printed in accordance with the original; I wouldn't dare to make any revisions. The essential principles of boxing have all been thoroughly detailed by those who came before me, so how could I presume to elaborate? If the wise and virtuous of the realm are able to follow this and seek out the principles and their benefits for body and mind, that will be a blessing for family and country.

Let us encourage each other in this pursuit.

—August 1948, Yang Shouzhong's respectful preface, at Yangshi

Taijiquan Form Sections

Section One: Taijiquan Beginning Form

This is the taijiquan posture for preparing to move. Stand in stillness *(li ding shi)*. The head must be upwardly aligned *(zheng zhi)*.

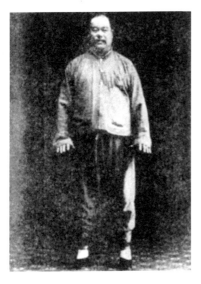

Figure 1

The intent is on the energy at the crown of the head *(yi han ding jin)*. The eyes look forward evenly. Contain the chest and draw up the back. You must not bow forward or lean backward. Sink the shoulders and drop the elbows. The fingertips of the two hands point forward; the palms face down. Loosen the waist and the *kua*. The two feet tread the ground, parallel, and separated to a distance equal to the shoulders. You must in particular secure the spirit of vitality within *(jingshen nei gu)*. The *qi* sinks to the *dantian*. Allow it to do so spontaneously *(yi ren ziran);* you must not force it *(bu ke qian qiang)*. I hold to my own stillness in order to deal with the other's movement; thus the inner and the outer are unified, essence and application are integrated. People all too easily neglect this posture, and really do not know the method of its practice or its application. It is all right here. One hopes that the student pays primary attention to this.

Translator's Comments

The first thing that strikes the reader about the description of the Beginning Form is that there is no description of the raising and lowering of the arms. The photo shows the position of the hands as they would be following the raising of the arms to shoulder height, then lowering them to the sides of the body. Could it be that the raising and lowering of the arms, so emblematic as the opening of the received form, was optional in earlier versions? An earlier form manual, Xu Yusheng's 1921 *Taijiquan shi tujie* (Illustrated Explanations of Taijiquan), also lacks a description of the raising of the arms. The emphasis here is clearly on the classical postural alignment prescriptions, the inner intent vital to taijiquan practice, and the stillness that balances movement.

Section Two: The *Peng* Method of Grasp Sparrow's Tail

Grasp Sparrow's Tail is the chief hand method of taijiquan's essence and application; that is, the so-called adhere, connect, stick, and follow *(nian, lian, tie, sui)* of push hands—to go back and forth

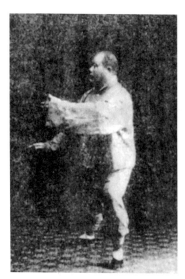

(wangfu) without separating or severing the connection *(bu li bu duan)*. Hence the figure of speech "Sparrow's Tail" refers to the hand and arm. Therefore we have the general term "Grasping the Sparrow's Tail." Its methods are four: Ward Off *(peng)*, Roll Back *(lu)*, Press *(ji)*, and Push *(an)*.

As for the method of Ward Off, from the Beginning Form, suppose an opponent directly facing me strikes at my chest with his left hand. I separate my right foot toward the right side, sitting solidly

Figure 2

22

on it. Then, raise the left foot, and take a step out to the front, bending the knee and sitting solidly on it. The rear leg extends straight. Consequently, the left is full and the right is empty.

At the same time, take the left hand and lift it up in front of the chest, with the heart of the palm facing in. The elbow drops slightly. Then, using my wrist to attach to the opponent's arm between the elbow and wrist, I use horizontal energy *(heng jin)* to ward off forward and upwardly *(peng qu)*. One must not show a stiff and wooden appearance; then, when the opponent's strength has already been shifted by me, his position becomes unstable of its own accord.

Translator's Comments

Yang Chengfu explains the name "Grasp Sparrow's Tail" *(lan que wei)*, describing it as the "chief hand," and he refers to the individual methods of Ward Off *(peng)*, Roll Back *(lu)*, Press *(ji)*, and Push *(an)* as subsets of Grasp Sparrow's Tail. The notion of "back and forth" *(wangfu* 往复*)*, or "to and fro," will appear again in the book in describing an interactive dynamic essential in push hands. The term *wangfu* appears in a line in Wu Yuxiang's "Mental Elucidation of the Thirteen Postures": "In going to and fro, there must be foldings and alternations."

Note that there is a change in voice from first person: "suppose an opponent directly facing me," to prescriptive voice: "take the left hand and lift it up." This shift in voice recurs throughout the book and most likely reflects a common phenomenon that occurs when someone is both demonstrating and explaining techniques to students.

There is some divergence of interpretation regarding the orientation of Yang's torso and face. Some Yang Style proponents learn the posture Ward Off Left with the torso facing more squarely toward the south. In his book, *Yang Chengfu Shi Taijiquan,* Yang Zhenji cites several authorities who learned from his father, noting that in their forms, "all have Left Ward

Off with the eyes looking in the direction of the left hand." He further remarks that

> According to the fighting methods handed down in the Yang family, it is necessary that the eyes focus in the direction towards which the left hand wards-off. Why, then, does the photo show the eyes looking toward the right side? It would seem now that at the time the photo was taken, the photographer made an error. (Yang Zhenji, *Yang Chengfu Shi Taijiquan,* pp. 25–26.)

Yang Zhenji does not elaborate on what the nature of the error was, but it could be that the photographer captured Yang Chengfu in a transitional movement, rather than in the precise ending posture for Ward Off Left.

Section Three: The *Lu* Method of Grasp Sparrow's Tail

From the previous posture, suppose the opponent uses his left hand to strike my ribs. I immediately step directly forward to the right front with my right foot, bending the knee and treading solidly. The left foot changes to empty. At the same time, my body also turns to face the right. The eyes, following, look out evenly. The right and left hands simultaneously turn over roundly and move toward the right front. The right hand is in front, the palm inclined toward the inside. The left hand is behind, the palm inclined toward the inside.

Turning to the point where the right palm is down and the left

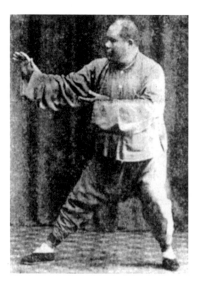

Figure 3

palm is facing up, I quickly adhere to the opponent's elbow joint with the side of my forearm. Inclining my left wrist, using the bone of the back of the wrist to stick to the wrist and back of the arm of the opponent, I incline it leftward and outward. The entire body sits on the left leg. The left foot is now full and the right foot is empty. If the opponent attacks at this time, I then turn him in before my chest. As the right side of the Roll Back engages, then the opponent's rooting strength is pulled up. His body also follows, and falls away at an incline!

Translator's Comments

The first paragraph of the *Lu Method* description is actually the description of Right Ward Off, but there is no explicit mention of Right Ward Off. The description of Roll Back does not begin until the second paragraph.

Section Four: The *Ji* Method of Grasp Sparrow's Tail

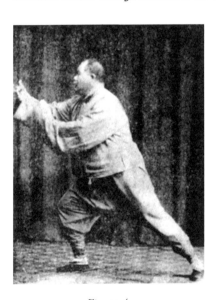

Figure 4

From the previous posture, suppose the opponent pulls back his arm. I then bend my right knee. The right foot becomes full, while the left leg extends straight. Extend the waist and lengthen toward him. Follow him and advance forward. The expression in the eyes is also delivered straight forward and upward. At the same time, quickly rotate the wrist of the right hand out. The palm of the left hand adheres along the right arm or wrist and advances forward, taking advantage of the opportunity provided by him pulling back his arm. Follow, and issue Press *(ji)* to him. Then the opponent will certainly be dropped smoothly!

Translator's Comments

The photo identified here (and throughout the book) as Press *(ji)* does not appear to show the left palm actually touching the right forearm. As such, the posture shown could in fact be Right Ward Off, but as noted above, there is no actual mention of Right Ward Off within the form descriptions.

Section Five: The *An* Method of Grasp Sparrow's Tail

From the previous posture, suppose the opponent, seizing the strategic advantage, applies Press to me from the left flank. With my

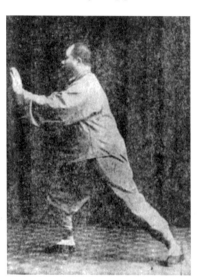

Figure 5

two wrists, I immediately apply lifting energy *(tijin)* from the left side upward, emptying the force of his Press. With fingers pointing upward, palms facing forward, sink the shoulders and drop the elbows. Seating the wrists and containing the chest, the entire body sits back on the left leg. Quickly use the two palms to push his elbow and wrist. Close in *(bi)* and push forward. Bending the right knee, sit solidly on it. Extend the left leg and waist while attacking forward. The expression in the eyes accords with the movement and is delivered forward from above. Then the opponent inclines backward and drops away!

Translator's Comments

The specific maneuver described for applying lifting energy (*tijin* 提勁) is not necessarily explicit in the solo form, but is a feature of push hands practice.

Section Six: Single Whip

From the previous posture, suppose an opponent comes from behind my body to strike me. I then shift my center of gravity *(zhongxin)* to the left foot, raise up the toes of the right foot, and turn to the left side, sitting solidly on the left leg. The left and right hands lift up on level with the shoulders, with the palms facing downward. Everything together follows the waist, and the movement swings left and right, back and forth, using the power of a steelyard's pivot. When the two hands again swing to the left, then collect the five fingers of the right hand, dropping them down and making a hook hand. At this moment, the left palm stops for an instant before the waist, forming an embrace with the hook hand, the heart of the palm facing upward. With the right foot in its original position, turn the body, rotating to the left rear. The left foot lifts up, stepping out to the left side. Bend the knee and sit solidly on the left leg as the right leg extends straight. The waist turns concurrently. The left hand draws in to the center, passing one's face, extending out as a palm toward the left. The heart of the palm faces out. Loosening the waist and the *kua*, close in *(bi)*

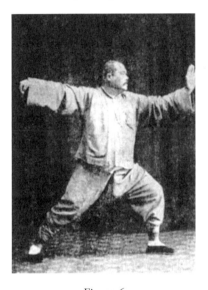

Figure 6

on the opponent's chest. Sink the shoulders, drop the elbows, and seat the wrists. The expression of the eyes follows the movement out to the front. If these movements are done with coordination, your opponent will certainly fall down.

Translator's Comments

There is no photo of Yang Chengfu performing the transition from Push to Single Whip, and there are varying interpretations within the Yang style of the footwork and hand positions within the transition itself. The narrative here clearly prescribes a shift of the weight to the left foot prior to turning the body to the left, but some Yang proponents teach this with a weighted pivot on the right foot. Yang's earlier book, *Taijiquan shiyongfa*, in fact clearly prescribes keeping the weight over the right leg for the leftward pivot. At the time Zheng Manqing edited the book, Yang may have changed the way he taught this pivot, or both ways may have been taught as alternates. The term "center of gravity" (*zhongxin* 重心) also did not appear in the earlier book, but appears twice in *Taijiquan tiyong quanshu*. It is not a traditional taijiquan term, but a neologism introduced into China along with Western concepts of mechanics and physics. It was easily assimilated into the modern taijiquan lexicon.

The terminology for "hook hand" here is not the usual term, but *diao zi shi*, literally, to make your hand into the shape of the *diao* 吊 character, one of whose meanings is "to suspend, to hang."

A more literal translation of the final phrase would be, "there is nobody who will not fall down easily" (*weiyou bu yingshou dao* 未有不應手倒). The phrase contains the compound *yingshou* 應手, literally, "respond/hand," which essentially means something that comes easily to hand. It is shorthand for *dexin yingshou* 得心應手, an expression about great skill, where the hand and mind work in concert. That phrase in turn came from the story of Wheelwright Pian in the *Zhuangzi,* who said of his woodworking skill, "Not too gentle, not too hard—you can get it in your hand and feel it in your mind. You can't put it into words, and yet there's a knack to it somehow." (Watson, *The Complete Works of Chuang Tzu,* p. 153.)

Section Seven: Raise Hands Upward

From the previous posture, suppose an opponent at my right flank comes to strike me. I then turn my body from the left back to the right. The left foot, following, moves in the turn to the right. The right foot lifts up and takes an advancing step toward the front. The heel of the foot lightly touches the ground; the toes of the foot suspend in emptiness. The whole body sits on the left leg. Contain the chest; pull up the back. Loosen the waist and look forward. At the same time, lift *(ti)* and close *(he)* the two hands toward the center. This is an instance of "closing energy" *(yi he jin).* The right hand is in front, and the left hand in back.

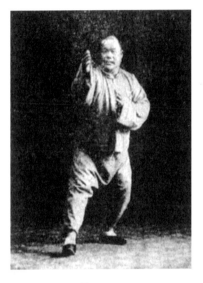

Figure 7

The two palms face each other, left and right. When the two wrists rise to the point where they join with the opponent's elbow and wrist, then you must contain and store the force, in order to wait in readiness for his changes. Or, I may also immediately turn my right palm to face upward and use the palm of my left hand to join with my right wrist and Press forth *(ji chu).* With regard to body method and foot method, this also has features similar to Press *(ji).*

Translator's Comments

The leftward turn of the body as described implies a weighted pivot on the left foot, since no shifting of weight is mentioned.

The containing of the force refers to a joint-lock application of Raise Hands Upward. To wait in readiness for the opponent's changes means that it is not necessary to follow through with the more destructive possibilities of the lock. The appropriate measure depends upon the action of the opponent.

The alternate application of Press may have taken place in the course of Yang's demonstration, in response to his demonstration partner evading or neutralizing the joint lock. The application of Press (or in Zheng Manqing's later form, Shoulder) is implied in the transition from Raise Hands Upward to White Crane Displays Wings.

Section Eight: White Crane Displays Wings

From the previous posture, suppose the opponent uses two hands to strike from my left side. I quickly draw back my right foot, then lift it up and step straight forward. Bend the knee slightly and sit solidly on the right leg. The body follows the right foot in turning simultaneously to face directly to the left. The left foot shifts to a point in front of the right foot, with the toes of the foot lightly touching the ground. The left hand concurrently closes with *(he yu)* the inside of the right forearm, then sinks to the abdomen. The right hand rises simultaneously with the sinking of the left hand, rising protectively to above the right temple, and spreads open *(zhan kai)* with the palm of

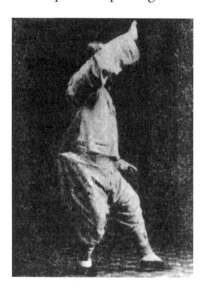

Figure 8

the right hand facing upward. The left hand as quickly proceeds downward, spreading open to the left beside the *kua*—the palm facing down. In this way, the opponent's strength is dissipated *(fensan)* and becomes disordered *(bu zheng)*.

Translator's Comments

The photo identified as White Crane Displays Wings is the same photo as that used for Retreat Astride Tiger. See my comments for that form in Section Eighty-Nine.

Section Nine: Left Brush Knee Twist Step

From the previous posture, suppose the opponent strikes from the left, with either a hand or a foot, at the middle or lower portion of my body. I let my body sink downward a bit, momen-

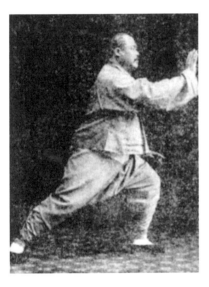

Figure 9

tarily placing the full strength upon the right leg. The left foot then lifts up and steps out to the front, then I bend the leg at the knee and sit solidly on it. The right leg, accordingly, stretches straight. The left hand concurrently turns up, arriving at the right front of the chest, then down to the left outside, brushing aside the hand or foot of the opponent. The right hand at once forms an upward-facing palm *(yang shou xin)*, then downward-hanging *(chui xia)*, turning now straight to the right rear and up to a point beside the ear. Extend the palm, with the heart of the palm facing forward. Sink the shoulders and drop the elbows. Seat the wrists, and loosen the waist into the forward advance. The expression of the eyes also accords with the forward motion. Push *(an)* forward toward the opponent's chest. The body and hands, each part must unite to produce one energy *(he cheng yi jin)*. The intention also extends boldly forward. This will ensure success.

Translator's Comments

The narrative here breaks this form section down into a) footwork, b) the action of the left hand, then c) the action of the right hand. The actions of all three must take place concurrently, but they were probably demonstrated separately for clarity of presentation.

Yang Zhenduo, in his book *Zhongguo Yang shi taiji,* lends clarity to the palm positions of the right hand, writing, "in transitioning from White Crane Displays Wings to Brush Knee Twist Step, the right arm circles down from above to in front of the thigh *(kua)*. The palm is up, the fingers toward the front, forming an upward palm. Continuing down in a circular arc, the palm turns toward the outside, the fingers pointing down, forming a downward-hanging palm. Now again the arm bends upward, turning the fingers to point up, the palm facing obliquely outward, forming a standing palm." (*Zhongguo Yang shi taiji*, p. 35.)

Note the important prescription that all parts of the body "unite to produce one energy" *(he cheng yi jin* 合成一勁). The term used for the mental intent that extends "boldly" forward is *yangchang* 揚長, which implies a proud bearing, with the head held high.

Section Ten: Hands Strum Pipa

From the previous posture, suppose the opponent, uses his right hand to strike my chest. I then contain my chest *(hanxiong)*, bend the right knee, and sit back solidly. The left foot accordingly shifts back and lifts, with the heel touching the ground, gathering and

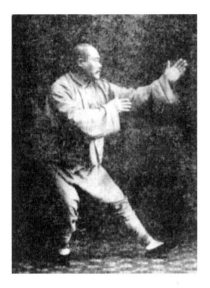

Figure 10

reserving its potential energy *(qi shi)*. The right hand concurrently draws in and closes, following along the opponent's wrist, and passing around and under it. I quickly use my wrist to stick to the opponent's wrist, then use my right hand to gather and join with the inside of his wrist to restrain and pull it to the right and downward. The left hand, also at the same time, advances forward and upward from the left, collecting and closing in. Using my palm and wrist, I stick to the opponent's elbow, making the shape of holding a *pipa*. At this instance, I am able to stand and fix my center of gravity; split *(lie)* with the left, pull down *(cai)* with the right, and reserve my power in order to observe his changes. This is called Hands Strum Pipa.

Translator's Comments

The phrase at the end of the sentence describing the action of the left foot — "gathering and reserving its potential energy" — was evidently added by Zheng Manqing. The term *qishi* 氣勢 can mean "momentum," a "gathering force," or an "imposing manner." The phrase "At this instance, I am able to stand and fix my center of gravity" was also evidently added by Zheng, and is the second occurrence of the term *zhongxin* 重心 (center of gravity) in the book.

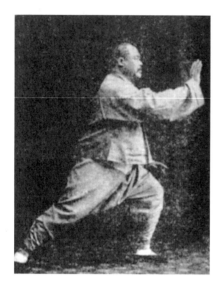

Figure 11

Section Eleven:
Left Brush Knee Twist Step

The application explanation for this posture is the same as for the ninth posture.

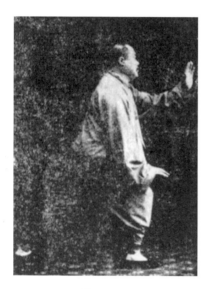

Figure 12

Section Twelve:
Right Brush Knee Twist Step

The application explanation for this posture is also the same as for the ninth posture, only left and right movements are reversed. Therefore they will not be repeated here. The reader may consult the above sections and will be able to understand.

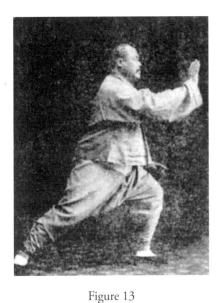

Figure 13

Section Thirteen:
Left Brush Knee Twist Step

The application and explanation are as above.

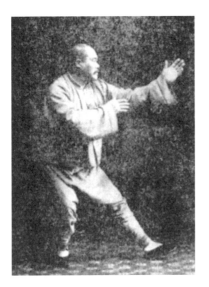

Figure 14

Section Fourteen:
Hands Strum Pipa

Posture is as explained above.

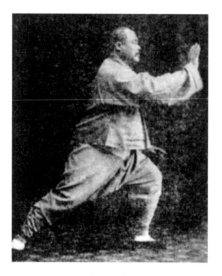

Section Fifteen:
Left Brush Knee Twist Step

The explanation of application is as above.

Translator's Comments

No details or explanations of the transitions for sections ten through sixteen are provided.

Figure 15

Section Sixteen: Advance Step, Deflect, Parry, and Punch

From the previous posture, suppose the opponent uses his right hand to strike. I then separate my left foot slightly out to the left side. The waist follows in the twisting turn to the left. The

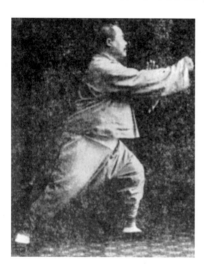

left hand then rotates and circles back to arrive beside the left ear, the palm downward. The right hand, relaxing at the wrist, follows the turning to arrive at the left mid-flank, forming a fist.

As the waist turns to the right, the wrist of the right hand turns out. Now this right fist follows, turning to arrive at the right lower flank. This is called "deflect" *(ban)*. At the same time, lift the right foot, and with the toes angled to the right, step

Figure 16

solidly. Loosen the waist and sink the *kua,* while the left hand strikes forward levelly from beside the left temple with an inclined palm. This is called "parry" *(lan).* The left foot concurrently lifts up and treads forward a step, sitting solidly. The right leg extends straight. The right fist then accords as one with the waist and leg as it strikes directly forward.

This, then, is the ingenious use of this fist *(quan).* It lies completely in neutralizing the incoming right fist of the other. First, using my right wrist, I stick to the opponent's right wrist, deflecting it from my left upper flank to the right lower flank. At this time, perhaps the opponent withdraws his arm and changes his stance. Then with my left hand coordinating with my step, I drive straight forward using open energy *(kaijin).* When I have parried his right hand, I then swiftly strike toward the opponent's chest. Then the opponent will be far too busy to avoid it, and will certainly serve as my target. This is the wonder of this fist: it lies completely in the unified method of deflect and parry.

Translator's Comments

The first two paragraphs describe the rather complex sequence of movements, while the third explains how the movements work in unbalancing an opponent and preparing him to "serve as my target." Some of the movement description gives an impression of sequential movements that are in fact synchronous. The leftward turn, for example, is all controlled by the turning of the waist. Yang Zhenji makes the role of the waist in this first sequence very explicit in his book, *Yang Chengfu Shi Taijiquan.* (p. 48). He writes:

The waist leads both hands and the turning of the ball of the left foot to the left. The toes of the left foot turn to point northeast, the left hand makes an outward rotation turning the palm to face upward, the right palm changes to a fist, the heart of the fist facing downward — the two hands follow the waist in their movements.

Section Seventeen: Like Sealing, As If Closing

From the previous posture, suppose the opponent uses his left hand to grasp my right fist. I then incline my left hand and thread under

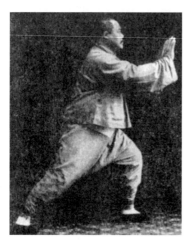

my right elbow, moving my palm protectively along the edge of my arm, attacking toward the opponent's left wrist. If the opponent wants to change hands in order to apply Push *(an)*, I then extend and open my right hand, pulling it toward my thorax to the point where the two palms are facing in and diagonally intersect like an oblique cross-shaped sealing tape *(fengtiao)*, preventing the opponent's hands from getting in. It is just like closing the door against a robber. This is why it is called "like sealing."

Figure 17

Concurrently, contain the chest and settle the *kua*, then separate the arms, changing so that the palms of the two hands apply Push *(an)* toward the opponent's elbow and wrist, making it impossible for him either to move to his advantage or to separate his arms. This is why it is called "as if closing." It is as if closing his door so that it cannot be opened.

Now, rapidly using "long energy" *(changjin)*, Push in accordance with the "an" posture. With eyes looking forward, the waist advances the attack, with the left leg bent at the knee and substantial, the right leg following the *kua* and extending straight, combining as one energy *(he yi jin)* and striking toward the opponent. This is the secret for getting it right.

Translator's Comments

This section not only describes the movements, but it also clarifies the name of the form, 如封似閉, which is often mistranslated as "apparent closure," or "withdraw and push," neither of which captures the separate actions of "sealing" (*feng* 封) and "closing" (*bi* 閉). The image used of "sealing tape" refers to *fengtiao* 封條, which were strips of red paper pasted across parcels, doors, crime scenes, etc., as seals. The term "long energy" (*changjin* 長勁) is movement that is soft, gradual, and extending forth with continuity. Yang Zhenji explains in *Yang Chengfu Shi Taijiquan*, "Long energy is the entire body from the feet to the legs, then the waist, expressed in the hands and arms, and strung together into one *jin*, extending the waist and lengthening forth to issue." (p. 30)

Section Eighteen: Cross Hands

From the previous posture, suppose there is an opponent striking downward from my right side. With my right arm, I swiftly

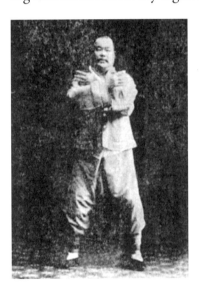

separate and extend upward to the right as my body turns to the right. The left foot closes with the right foot. The two hands spread from above, returning from below to join with one another to connect and form a cross shape. The entire body sits on the left foot. The right foot lifts up, collecting in to the left a half step. The two feet tread straight, as in the Beginning Form. This is at once opening and closing energy *(yi kai yi he jin)*. When I use opening energy to separate the opponent's hands, perhaps he just then takes advantage of my weak point and makes a surprise attack toward my chest. Therefore I join my two hands to produce closing energy

Figure 18

(yi he jin). At this time the hearts of the two palms face in, and I ward off *(peng zhu)* the opponent's arm. If the opponent changes to a two-hand Push, I then use my two hands to separate the opponent's hands from the inside to the right and left. The palms can face up or down — either will do. However, while forming the Cross Hands, you must at the same time slightly loosen the knees and waist, and sink downward. Then, the force coming from the opponent will dissipate itself!

Translator's Comments

Although it only appears as a named posture three times in the taijiquan set, Cross Hands occurs in many transitional movements and is incorporated into most of the kicks. The earliest published Yang taijiquan manual, Xu Yusheng's 1921 *Taijiquan shi tujie* (Illustrated Explanations of Taijiquan), highlights many occurrences of the posture that are not made explicit in the received form. In his section on Cross Hands, Xu wrote, "In those cases where the transition between two linked forms is not smooth, you can always add Cross Hands to assist in joining them." Interestingly, the line drawing for the posture in Xu's book shows the arms in a higher position than in Yang Chengfu's photo, with the ulnas turned forward and the wrists crossing above the forehead.

Yang Chengfu's narrative here shows the great potential in using Cross Hands to adapt to changing circumstances.

Section Nineteen: Embrace Tiger, Return to Mountain

From the previous posture, suppose an opponent draws near from behind to strike at my right side. With no time to distinguish whether he is using his hand or his foot, I quickly turn the waist, separating and opening the two hands. Take a step out to the right, bending the knee and sitting solidly over the right leg. The left leg extends straight. The right hand follows the turning of the waist toward the right, brushing at the height of the opponent's waist. Turning back from the "embrace" *(bao)*, the left hand also quickly

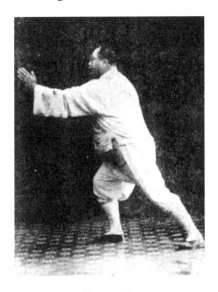

Figure 19a

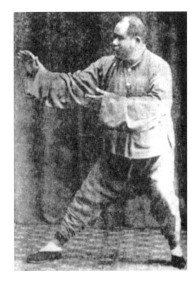

Figure 19b: Embrace Tiger,
Return to Mountain, *Lu* Form

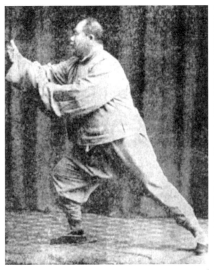

Figure 19c: Embrace Tiger,
Return to Mountain, *Ji* Form

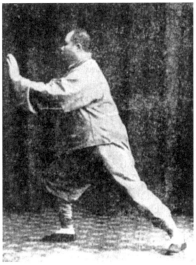

Figure 19d: Embrace Tiger,
Return to Mountain, *An* Form

follows, pushing *(an)* forward toward him. Therefore, the right hand first uses the covering wrist *(fu wan)* to brush forth, then turns and draws back using a raised palm *(yang zhang)*.

When doing the Embrace Tiger form, suppose the opponent's hands and feet are extremely fast, and that I am unable to hold on, but can only brush him aside or push him. Then the opponent will come back, changing to strike with his left hand. I then use the *lu* form to roll him back.

The remaining three forms of Grasp Sparrow's Tail proceed as explained above.

Translator's Comments

In this section, the "demonstration narrative" is quite evident. Again there is a shift in voice from first person to prescriptive, and one can vividly imagine Yang engaging a partner and showing the application possibilities.

The photo supplied seems to show Yang in an east-west orientation, but this section, including the Grasp Sparrow's Tail movements *Lu, Ji,* and *An,* actually proceeds to the northwest.

Section Twenty: Observe Fist Under Elbow

From the previous form, if an opponent comes to strike from the rear, I then turn my body—the movement is similar to the turning of the body in the prior Single Whip form. You may consult and use it. Then, just before the body is about to rotate to face squarely east, the left foot steps straight forward solidly. Then the right foot, with the toes toward the right front, steps forward a half-step. As the right foot becomes full, the left foot then rises up—the toes lift upward. The two hands are level with the shoulders, turning in concert with the body toward the left. At this time, immediately use the wrist of the left hand to open out levelly to connect with the opponent's right wrist, pushing toward his right, until he is driven to lose his central equilibrium. Now let the fingers of the hand drop down, hem in the opponent's wrist, and coil in

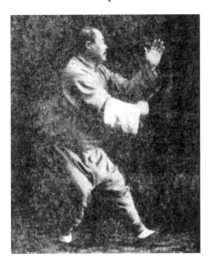

a small circle to the inside. The right hand concurrently moves leftward, connecting with his left hand, adhering from above. Thus the opponent's left and right hands are both contained, and he loses his orientation. Now I use my left wrist to raise his right wrist. My right hand swiftly forms a fist, turning and arriving beneath my left elbow, the tiger's mouth *(hukou)* facing up, in order to reserve its power

Figure 20

(xu qi shi), meet the opportunity, then issue. The opponent will fall in an instant. This is called Observe Fist Under Elbow.

Translator's Comments

In this sequence, having caused the opponent to "lose his central equilibrium" (*shique zhongding* 失却中定), Yang demonstrates his complete control and containment of the attacker, and his readiness to strike if necessary.

The posture name *zhou di kan chui* 肘底看捶 is translated literally as "Observe Fist Under Elbow." In Xu Yusheng's *Taijiquan shi tujie,* he wrote that the word *kan* 看 carries the meaning of the compound *kanshou* 看守, which means "to guard" or "to watch." This opens up several possible meanings for the form name, such as "guarding fist under elbow," "guarded fist under elbow," and the like. The notion of standing guard or being watchful suggests a reserving or storing up of power, only to be issued when the situation calls for it and the opportunity is right.

Section Twenty-One: Step Back Dispatch Monkey

From the preceding posture, suppose an opponent firmly grasps my left wrist or forearm with his right hand, and also uses his left hand to lift my right fist. Hence I am initially under his control. Just when it seems I can't display my skill, I immediately rotate my left palm up, and using sinking energy *(chenjin),* loosening my waist and *kua,* draw it back toward the left rear. The left foot also retreats a step, bending at the knee and sitting solid. The right foot changes to empty, then the opponent's gripping strength is suddenly lost. The right hand simultaneously separates and opens to the rear, and at the point when he loses his gripping strength, immediately pushes forward. Although this form retreats a step, it can still dispatch the opponent's energy. Hence it is named Step Back Dispatch Monkey. Its essentials are in particular the loosening of the shoulders *(song jian)* and the sinking of the *qi.*

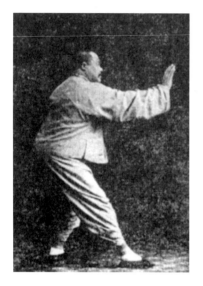

Figure 21

Translator's Comments

The interjection, "Just when it seems I can't display my skill," is an amusing setup for the reversal in fortunes the opponent is about to experience. It is also a commentary on the meaning of the form's name, *dao nian hou* 倒撵猴. The word *dao* 倒 can mean "to back up," "reverse," or "invert," but it can also mean "contrary to expectation." Hence the statement, "Although this form retreats a step, it can still dispatch the opponent's energy." One is reminded of the English phrase "to turn the tables" on someone.

Note the careful explanation of the timing involved. It is just at the point where the opponent "loses his gripping strength" that one applies the push.

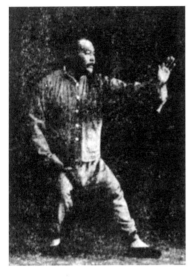

Figure 22

Section Twenty-Two: Step Back Dispatch Monkey, continued

The additional left and right forms of Step Back Dispatch Monkey are the same in intent. The body method, footwork, and posture are all identical. In practice one may retreat three, five, or seven steps. All of these are fine as long as one ends with the right hand in the forward position.

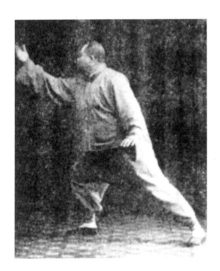

Figure 23

Section Twenty-Three: Flying Obliquely

From the previous form, if an opponent comes from the right side to strike my upper body, or uses strength to pin down my right forearm or wrist, I immediately take advantage of the situation, sink downward, close *(he)*, and store up energy *(xu jin)*. Thereupon I separate and spread my right hand to the upper right corner, using opening energy *(kaijin)* to strike obliquely. Simultaneously, I step out with the right foot, bending the knee and sitting solidly on the right leg. It resembles a posture of flying obliquely. The intent should reflect the name of the posture.

Translator's Comments

Yang's admonition to "take advantage of the situation" (*chengshi* 乘勢) clearly illustrates the importance of responding to and using the energy of an attacker to one's own advantage. In this case, the opponent's movement is neutralized by directing it downward to the left prior to the oblique rightward strike.

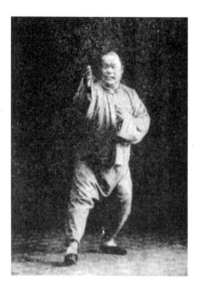

Section Twenty-Four:
Raise Hands Upward

This is the same as Section Seven.

Figure 24

46

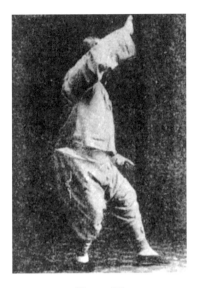

Figure 25

Section Twenty-Five:
White Crane Displays Wings
This is the same as Section Eight.

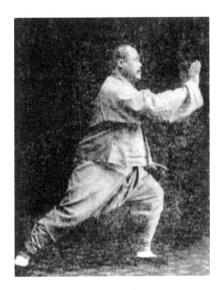

Figure 26

Section Twenty-Six:
Brush Knee Twist Step
This is the same as Section Nine.

Section Twenty-Seven: Needle at Sea Bottom

From the previous form, suppose the opponent uses his right hand to pull my right wrist. I then bend my right elbow and sit over

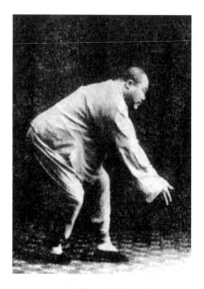

my right foot. Turn the waist, lifting back, with the right palm facing toward the left. The left foot also follows it in drawing back; the toes of the foot touch the ground. If the opponent still has not released my hand, and still wants to take advantage and strike me, I then let my right wrist follow the force with a loosening movement, folding the waist and sinking downward. The gaze of the eyes is forward. The fingertips hang down. The movement's intent is like that of a needle probing the sea bottom. At this moment, though he may want to pull or struggle, all of this going to and fro will become as one continuous strength, and he will unexpectedly meet with defeat. Then his rooting strength will sever itself. This will make it convenient for me to take advantage of his emptiness, to advance, and strike.

Figure 27

Translator's Comments

The "to and fro" (*wangfu* 往复) refers to a dynamic that develops within the whole sequence, including the following form, Fan Through Back. The initial rearward/upward pull of the right hand establishes a connection—a hooking up with the opponent's strength. Once the connection has been established, one then goes in the direction of his strength. The opponent's own persistence in hanging on brings the result: "his rooting strength will sever itself."

What does it mean that the to-and-fro exchanges become "one continuous strength" (*yi zhi li* 一直力)? If one were to strenuously resist the opponent at any point in this scenario, or use strength forcefully against his movements, it would add force to a situation where there is already force. There would, so to speak, be "two strengths." Since the opponent is using force, there is already strength available. The matter at hand is: What will become of this strength? By linking up with the opponent's strength, it becomes "one continuous strength," with one person in control of the situation.

Section Twenty-Eight: Fan Through Back

From the preceding posture, suppose the opponent again strikes, using his right hand. I then lift my right hand upward from the

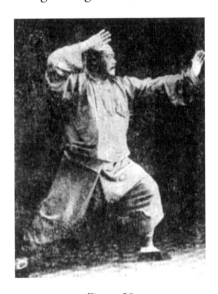

forward position to arrive beside my right temple, turning the palm to face outward, by this means supporting the energy of the opponent's right hand. The left hand simultaneously lifts in front of the chest, bursting forth *(chong kai)* with the palm. A continuous energy thrusts forth toward the opponent's flank. Sink the shoulders, drop the elbows, seat the wrists, and loosen the waist. The left foot concurrently steps toward

Figure 28

the front. Bend the knee and sit solidly on the left leg. The toes point forward. The vision follows the left hand and looks forward. The right leg coordinates with the waist and *kua* to extend the energy *(jin)* and send it forth. The *jin* actually issues from the back.

The two arms spread open *(zhan kai)*. You want the fan to connect through the back. Then you will be undefeatable.

Translator's Comments

"The left hand simultaneously lifts in front of the chest, bursting forth *(chong kai* 沖開) with the palm. A continuous energy thrusts forth toward the opponent's flank." This rather vivid language describes the trajectory of the left palm toward the rib cage of the opponent. I'm not aware of the verb combination *chongkai* having any technical martial art meaning. Here it is just descriptive of the manner in which the palm strikes forth, *chong* 沖 having overtones of "flowing," "flooding," "flushing," or like a dam bursting. The "continuous energy" *(zhi li* 直力) means strength that is both "direct, straight forward," and "continuous, uninterrupted." That is, it is a continuous movement throughout the whole body (opening out through the spine), not just of the arm itself. This can take the form of a disabling blow to the opponent, or it can merely make contact and add to his impetus, causing him to soar backward.

Section Twenty-Nine: Turn Body and Strike

From the preceding form, suppose an opponent comes from behind to strike my spine, back, or flank. I then turn on my left foot to the right, sitting solidly on it. The right foot changes to empty. The waist follows the turn to face squarely to the south. The right hand concurrently makes a fist, passing a moment before the chest, between the left flank and armpit. The palm of the left hand closes in an upward direction to protect the left temple. Immediately the right fist casts outward in an upward rotation from the radius of the elbow, intersecting with the opponent's hand, using sinking energy *(chenjin)* to fold it over to my right flank. At the same time, my left hand comes from my left side, swiftly striking toward the opponent's face, causing him to become utterly dazed and confused.

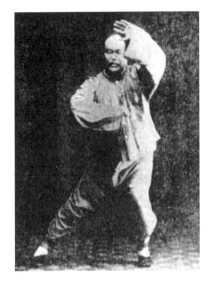
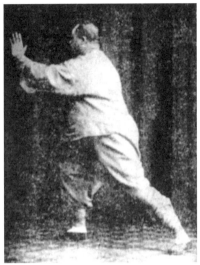

Figure 29a   Figure 29b

Translator's Comments

The form explanation here seems incomplete. The footwork is described up to the point depicted in the first photo, but there is no description of stepping out with the right foot to complete the 180° turn from Fan Through Back.

The initial rightward turn as described implies a weighted pivot on the left leg, but some Yang proponents advocate shifting the weight off the leg prior to the pivot.

The word *pie* 撇 in the form name refers to the casting out of the right back-fist, and its slanted trajectory across the torso, rather like the slanted stroke in calligraphy 丿 also named *pie*.

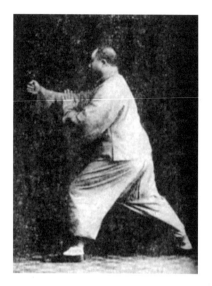

Figure 30

Section Thirty: Advance Step, Deflect, Parry, and Punch

The application is identical to Section Sixteen.

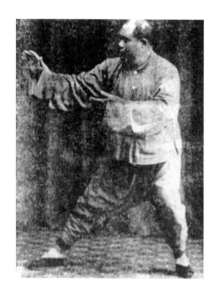

Figure 31

Section Thirty-One: Step Up, Grasp Sparrow's Tail

For Roll Back, Press, and Push, consult Sections Three through Five.

Translator's Comments

There is no mention of Ward Off in the Step Up, Grasp Sparrow's Tail section here, but there is a Right Ward Off in this section of the received form.

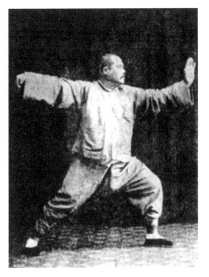

Figure 32

Section Thirty-Two:
Single Whip

This is identical to Section Six.

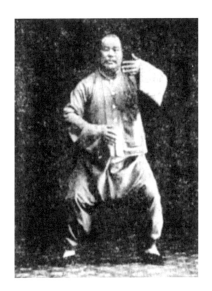

Figure 33

Section Thirty-Three:
Cloud Hands

From the preceding posture, suppose the opponent strikes with his right hand toward my chest or flank from the right front. I then let my right hand drop downward, with the palm toward the inside. Then I let the upper edge of my wrist come into contact with the lower part of the opponent's wrist, across to the left, then upward and revolving again toward the right, again rotating downward and moving leftward, drawing a large circle. This is like a cloud moving through the sky, continuously without end. The left hand, in like manner, follows in dropping down, with the palm facing down, tracing downward and rotating upward. The application is the same as for the right hand. The body also accords with the right hand in twisting and turning, and the vision follows the hands and wrists, coordinating the circles. The right foot shifts a half-step to the left, becoming full. The left foot then steps out a step to the left, forming a horse-riding stance *(qi ma shi)*. At this time, the two hands are directly aligned in their movement before the chest and the navel. Then the right foot again changes to empty, sitting in a half-step toward the left. Now continue the movement through the second form. However, in the course of changing from empty to full, and in alternating of circles, by no means should there be any instance of hollows and protuberances, or any intermittence. The subtle usage of this form lies entirely in the turning of the waist and *kua*. Then you will be able to draw out the opponent's rooting strength with a smooth turning out of the wrist. Students must be aware of these details.

Translator's Comments

No specific guidelines are given for the number of repetitions, but most modern adherents prescribe three, five, or seven. The Cloud Hands section presents particular challenges for written description, and the description here is frankly rather vague. The problem, again, has to do with trying to portray simultaneous movements with sequential language. Any shortcomings in the written depiction of body mechanics are compensated for by highlighting the need to turn the waist and *kua,* and the "drawing out of the opponent's rooting strength" *(qian dong di zhi gen li)* with "a smooth turning out of the wrist" *(yingshou fan chu).*

54

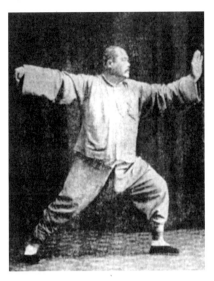

Figure 34

Section Thirty-Four:
Single Whip

This is identical to Section Six.

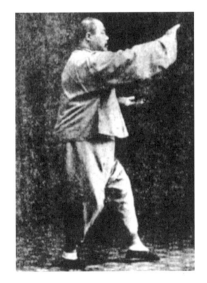

Figure 35

Section Thirty-Five:
High Pat on Horse

From the Single Whip posture, suppose the opponent evades and coils from beneath my left wrist with his left hand, probing toward the right side of my body. I follow, letting my left wrist drop with loosening energy *(song jin)*. With the palm facing upward, I fold it against the opponent's wrist and pluck *(cai)* it back in toward my chest, as in the illustration. The left foot simultaneously lifts back, the toes touching the ground. Loosen the waist and contain the chest. The right knee bends slightly as you sit solidly on the right leg. At the same time, quickly bring the right hand from the rear to circle forward and upward, stretching the palm toward the opponent's face. The eyes look forward. The slight raising of the spine and back has the intention both of stretching and drawing upward, and advancing forward *(tan ba qian jin)*.

Translator's Comments

Conventionally translated "High Pat on Horse," the Chinese name *gao tan ma* 高探馬 calls upon imagery that may reflect special familiarity with matters equestrian. The verb *tan* means "to test, to put out a feeler, to explore, spy, scout," as well as the physical motion of "stretching forth." All of these connotations apply in the posture, which requires a rising up and a stretching forth. There is, incidentally, a compound, *tanma* 探馬, which means a mounted scout. Xu Yusheng evokes this in his explanation of the form name: "The body towers upward, reaching outward to the front, rather like the appearance of being mounted on a horse, with the body reaching forward." (*Taijiquan shi tujie*, p. 28.)

Section Thirty-Six: Right Separate Feet, with Roll-Back Form

From the previous posture, suppose the opponent uses his left hand to connect with my forward-stretching right wrist. I apply pressure to the opponent's left elbow with my right wrist, dropping my elbows and sinking my shoulders. I then roll back the opponent's left arm toward my left side, with my left wrist simultaneously sticking to his left wrist. With the left palm facing down, there is a hidden application of pull down *(an shi cai jin)*. At the same time, the left foot steps forward to the left side a half-step, becoming full.

The waist faces obliquely toward the left. Following, lift the right foot upward, and kick levelly and directly toward the opponent's left rib cage, with the toes and the back of the foot. Concurrently,

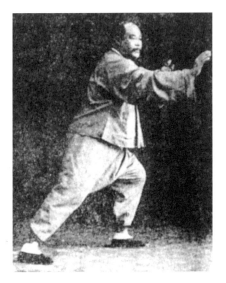
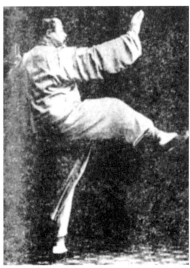

Figure 36a: Right Separate Feet, *Lu* Form   Figure 36b

the two palms stand up obliquely, separating and opening toward the left and right, on level with the shoulders, to balance the separating form of the legs. The eyes also follow and watch the right hand. Contain the chest and pull up the back. Concentrate the strength from the foot. Then the opponent will be unable to sustain his position.

Translator's Comments

In Sections Thirty-Six and Thirty-Seven, I have added the words "with Roll-Back Form" to the section heads. Both include the front-weighted Roll Back photos identified as right and left Roll-Back form, respectively. As prescribed here, the Roll Back is clearly a prerequisite to the kick.

The "hidden application" (*an shi* 暗施) mentioned here refers to a rotation of the forearm at the end of the Roll Back, so that the left palm can apply the *cai* technique to further unbalance the opponent.

Although the description includes the separating of the palms that accompanies the kick, there is no mention of the Cross-Hands form that precedes the separating.

Section Thirty-Seven: Left Separate Feet, with Roll-Back Form

The functionality is identical to the right side form above, only left and right exchange places.

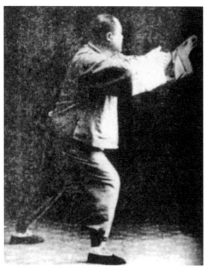
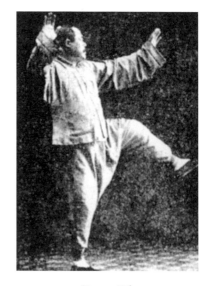

Figure 37a: Left Separate Feet, *Lu* Form   Figure 37b

Section Thirty-Eight: Turn Body and Kick with Heel

From Left Separate Feet, suppose an opponent uses his right hand to strike me from behind. I immediately turn my body squarely to the left. Contain the chest and pull up the back. Loosen the waist, and in particular you must allow an intangible and lively energy to lift the crown of the head *(xu ling ding jin)*. The left

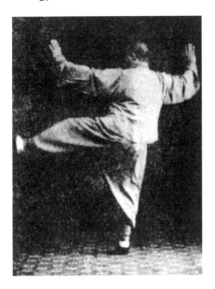

leg is suspended and lifted. Following the turning of the waist, the toes drop down. When the right leg becomes firmly established, the left foot then kicks toward the opponent's abdomen, using the heel. The toes of the foot point up. As the two hands follow the turning of the waist, they collect inward from the prior outward position. The palms, in accord with the left foot kicking forth, lift to the left and right sides, separating and opening level with the shoulders. The gaze of the eyes follows the fingertips of the left hand. Firmly establish your rooting strength, then the opponent will surely have a reactive response in his legs and will fall back of his own accord!

Figure 38

Translator's Comments

The turn here is a 180° counter-clockwise pivot, with the resulting heel kick "squarely" to the west. Although the form named is conventionally translated Turn Body, Kick with Heel, the verb *deng* 蹬 is not necessarily well-served by the translation "kick." The word *deng* really means "to tread," with the sole of the foot. The raised leg movements in taijiquan are not necessarily kicks in the conventional sense of a power kick. They certainly can be applied in that manner, but they can also simply make contact with an opponent's unbalanced body, adding just enough force to send him or her soaring back.

The above interpretation of this kick accounts for the translation of the sentence, "Then the opponent will surely have a reactive response in his legs and will fall back of his own accord!" The wording is ambiguous, and it is unclear whether *ying tui* 應腿 refers to the opponent's response to the kicking leg, or to a response in his own legs as he stumbles backward. The fact that he falls back "of his own accord" (*zi yang* 自仰) could imply the latter case.

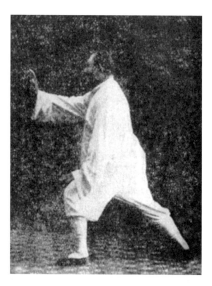

Figure 39

Section Thirty-Nine: Left Brush Knee

This is performed as above.

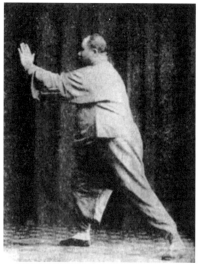

Section Forty:
Right Brush Knee

This is performed as above.

Figure 40

Section Forty-One: Advance Step, Plant Punch

From the previous posture, suppose the opponent again kicks with his left foot. I immediately use my left hand to follow the force

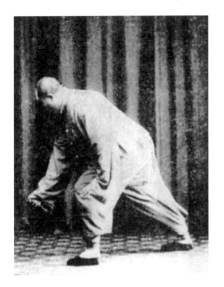

of his leg, brushing it to my left, then he will certainly fall toward the left. At the same time, I advance forward a step with my left foot, bending that knee and sitting solidly. The right hand follows, forming a fist, and punches either toward the opponent's waist or shin — both are possible. This is called planting punch *(zai chui)*. At this time, the right leg extends straight. The sinking of the waist and *kua* achieves a balanced but bent form. The chest is contained and the eyes look forward. In particular, I must hold to my center ground *(shou wo zhongtu)*. This is essential.

Figure 41

Translator's Comments

In the sentence "I immediately use my left hand to follow the force of his leg. . . ," the photo reproduction of *Taijiquan tiyong quanshu* in the back of Yang Zhenji's book shows a handwritten correction of the character "right" to "left." I have followed the emendation.

Xu Yusheng writes that the "planting punch" *(zai chui* 栽捶) in the name refers to the fact that it resembles the form of someone planting seedlings in the earth.

The "balanced but bent form" refers to the body's folding at the pelvis, but still remaining aligned and balanced.

The wording "I must hold to my center ground" *(shou wo zhongtu* 守我中土) does not appear in Yang's earlier book,

Taijiquan shiyongfa, so it may have been added by Zheng Manqing. The reference to "central earth" 中土 is unusual, and is probably an idiomatic phrase for another Taiji term, "central equilibrium" (*zhongding* 中定), which is association with earth. The phrase *shou zhongtu* appears in the body of taiji texts known as the "Yang Forty," in a short text titled "Training Methods for Sparring, or Holding the Central Earth." (See Douglas Wile, *Lost T'ai-chi Classics from the Late Ch'ing Dynasty,* pp. 67–68, p. 137.) The phrase may have been inspired by the idea of "holding the center" (*shouzhong* 守中), appearing in chapter 5 of the *Daodejing.* Yang Chengfu's first son's sobriquet was this same *Shouzhong.*

Section Forty-Two: Obverse Turn Body and Strike

From the previous posture, suppose there is another opponent coming to strike with a fist from behind me. I then turn my body toward the right and to the rear, sitting solidly on the left foot. The right leg lifts up and steps forward a half-step, with the right fist simultaneously lifting and casting squarely out to the east, with

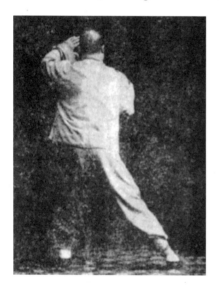
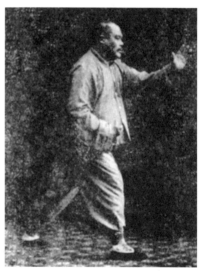

| Figure 42a | Figure 42b |

the back of the fist sinking down. One can either use this to fold up the opponent's elbow, or apply the hidden application of pull-down energy *(an yong cai jin)*—both are possibilities. The left hand simultaneously follows the right fist and splits *(lie)* out toward the opponent's face with the palm in order to augment the casting power of the right fist. The body must follow, and then you will make headway in obtaining the advantage *(de shi)*.

Translator's Comments

The prior Turn Body and Strike, at Section Twenty-Nine, which turns from east to west, is named *pie shen chui*, while this section is named *fan shen pie shen chui*. I've translated this as Obverse Turn Body and Strike, since it turns from west to east.

Once again, a weighted pivot on the left foot is implied in the narrative, but it is ambiguous.

The "hidden application" would require a rotation of one's right forearm to turn an open palm to make contact with the opponent's wrist.

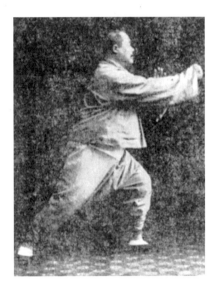

Section Forty-Three: Advance Step, Deflect, Parry, and Punch

This is similar to Section Sixteen, above.

Figure 43

Section Forty-Four: Right Kick with Heel

From the previous posture, suppose the opponent uses his left hand to push my right arm toward my left side. At this time,

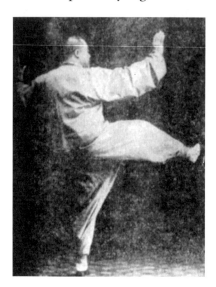

Figure 44

I let my right wrist follow the force of his movement and coil beneath the opponent's wrist from the right to the left, then split open. [The toes of the left foot, meanwhile, have turned slightly to the left. Sitting solidly on the left leg, the torso also follows through, turning directly toward the left.] My two hands separate and open, coordinating with the foot. The waist and *kua* sink down. The vision follows, looking toward the front. At the same time, the right foot kicks *(deng)* squarely out.

Translator's Comments

The bracketed material was at the end of this section in the original, but I have placed it in what would be the logical movement sequence. Still, the sequence as presented is problematic, since the "splitting open" *(lie kai)* of the right arm is concurrent with the separating of the two hands. Again, there is a Cross Hands form prior to the separating out of the hands in the received form, but it is not explicitly described in the narrative.

Section Forty-Five: Left Hit Tiger Form

From the previous form, suppose an opponent on my left strikes forward using his left hand. I let my right foot lower down and align it evenly with the left. The left and right hands follow the turning of the body toward the left side. The left foot steps out

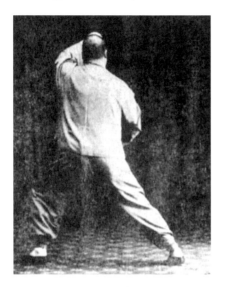

Figure 45

toward the rear, bending at the knee and sitting solid. The right foot changes to empty, approximately forming an oblique horse-riding form. The face is toward the corner of the square. The two hands simultaneously swing—forming fists—down and toward the left in unison. Then, use the right fist to restrain the opponent's left wrist, pulling down *(cai)* and toward my left side, and aligned on an axis with the heart. The left fist moves left, rotating outward and up, turning until it arrives next to my left temple. The heart of the fist faces out. It can quickly hit either the opponent's head or back. This form turns a retreat into an advance, suddenly opening, suddenly closing. The intent is to contain ferocity, hence the name, Hit Tiger Form.

Translator's Comments

There is some confusion, and variance of interpretation, regarding the directionality of the two Hit the Tiger forms. If one takes the floor patterns as a guide, the photos of Yang Chengfu depict a cardinal north-south orientation (with the right form depicted as a side view). Yet the written narrative describes a step "out to the rear," resulting in a posture facing "the corner of the square." Both Fu Zhongwen's and Yang Zhenji's form instructions prescribe the forms as aligned on the bias, with the Left Hit Tiger facing northwest, and the Right Hit Tiger facing southeast. Yang Zhenduo, however, teaches the sequence to the cardinal north and south directions. Yang Chengfu's earlier book, *Taijiquan shiyongfa,* does not contain the wording about stepping out to the rear or facing the corner, but rather describes facing to "the left side of the square" (*mian xiang zuo zheng fang* 面向左正方).

Zheng Manqing evidently made some changes to the original *Taijiquan shiyongfa* instructions. The verb "swing" (*dang* 盪) describing the sweep of the arms to the left, for example, does not appear in the earlier version. The envoi statements about turning a retreat into an advance, and the form name reflecting ferocity, were also added. The formulation "suddenly opening, suddenly closing" *(hu kai hu he)* resembles the phrase "suddenly hidden, suddenly appearing" *(hu yin hu xian)* from the "Taijiquan Treatise," but this way of expressing contrasts is common in Chinese.

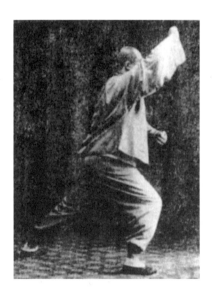

Figure 46

Section Forty-Six:
Right Hit Tiger Form

From the previous posture, suppose an opponent comes to strike me with his right hand from my right rear flank. I then lift up my right foot, stepping out to the right side, bending my knee and sitting solid. This approximates a right horse-riding form. The waist follows, turning toward the right front direction. The left leg changes to empty. The two fists

concurrently follow toward the right, turning in circles and forming Right Hit Tiger Form. The functionality is the same as for the
left form. I hope you will refer to it.

Section Forty-Seven: Turn Body, Right Kick with Heel

This is similar to Section Forty-Four. The directions of left and
right may change.

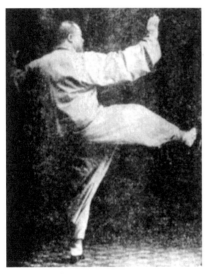

Translator's Comments

It is not clear what the ratio-
nale may have been for adding
the remark "The directions of
left and right may change."
The demonstration may have
included an alternate pos-
sibility of a left kick, but the
received form is as pictured.

Figure 47

Section Forty-Eight: Twin Gusts Penetrate the Ears

From the previous form, suppose the opponent comes from my
right flank, striking with both hands. I then shift the toes of
my left foot, turning slightly to the right, still standing stable.
The right foot is at the same time suspended during the turn to
the right, with the knee lifted upward, the toes dropped downward. The torso concurrently follows the turning, arriving to face
directly into the corner. Swiftly move the backs of the two hands

downward from above, causing the opponent's two wrists to separate out and fold back. Then I move my two hands upward from below, forming fists. Using the opposing tiger's mouths of the two fists, strike piercingly toward the opponent's two ears. The right foot simultaneously drops toward the front and down, changing to full. The torso, then and only then, expresses the intent of advancing an attack.

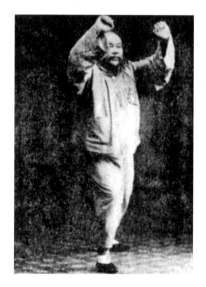

Translator's Comments

This form is sometimes named Twin Peaks Strike the Ears. The characters for "peak" 峰 and "wind" 風 are both pronounced *feng*. The one used here is the one meaning "wind," which I've translated as "gust." Xu Yusheng wrote in *Taijiquan shi tujie* that the name means "nimble as the wind."

Figure 48

Section Forty-Nine: Left Heel Kick

From the previous posture, suppose there is an opponent coming on my left flank to strike at my rib cage. I quickly use my left hand to stick to the back of the opponent's right hand, drawing it in, then splitting *(lie)* open. The right foot makes a slight shift to the right. The left foot at the same time lifts upward toward the front, kicking toward the opponent's ribs or abdomen. The remainder is like Turn Body, Kick with Heel.

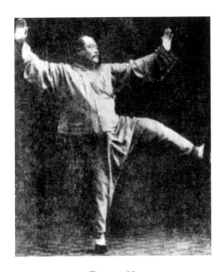

Figure 49

Translator's Comments
The prescription to draw the opponent's hand in, prior to splitting open, implies the Cross-Hands position of the received form (not depicted).

Section Fifty: Turn Body, Kick with Heel

Connecting with the previous form, if an opponent comes to strike from behind my back to my left, I quickly spin my body in an about-face to the right rear. At the same time the body is turning, the left foot draws in and is suspended in the turn to the right, toward the front. During this turn, the ball of the right foot serves as the pivot *(shuji)* for the spinning of the whole body. When the two hands close and gather in following the body's turn, swiftly use the wrist of the right hand to stick to the opponent's forearm, coming down

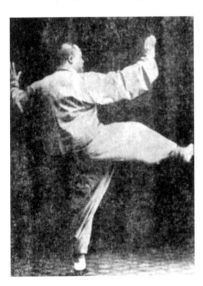

Figure 50

from above and splitting out *(lie)* toward the right. The right foot simultaneously lifts up to kick *(deng)* his flank or abdomen as the right and left hands separate and open accordingly toward the front and rear.

Translator's Comments

The word *shuji* 樞機 is an unusual word choice for "pivot" in this passage, as it tends to refer to something more abstract than a physical pivot point. Evidently, this is another sign of Zheng Manqing's influence on the text. In fact, in the earlier section narrative version in *Taijiquan shiyongfa,* the word used is a more common term for pivot: *shuniu* 樞扭. It is quite probable that in using the term *shuji* Zheng was inspired by the source text for that term, which is the *Xici* commentary of the *Book of Changes.* There we find the sentence "Words and actions are the door hinge and crossbow trigger of the noble man." (Richard John Lynn, trans., *The Classic of Changes,* p. 18.) The word *shu* 樞 is literally "door hinge," and *ji* 機 is "trigger." But as a compound, *shuji* came to mean something like "the controlling action." We know that Zheng was closely familiar with the *Xici* and enjoyed drawing upon its words and imagery. The imagery of a hinge has perennial philosophical significance in the Chinese tradition. An example is the notion of the *daoshu* 道樞 (hinge, or pivot of the *dao*), found in the second chapter of *Zhuangzi,* where it is described, "A state in which 'this' and 'that' no longer find their opposites is called the hinge of the Way. When the hinge is fitted into the socket, it can respond endlessly." (Watson, *The Complete Works of Chuang Tzu,* p. 40.) Perhaps Zheng Manqing, by this subtle choice of words, meant to make reference to the inner, psychological pivot, which is every bit as vital as the mechanical pivot described.

The Cross Hands component of this section is more clearly described here than it is for some of the other kicks.

I've followed Yang Zhenji's emendation changing "left" to "right" for the direction of the *lie* action of the right hand.

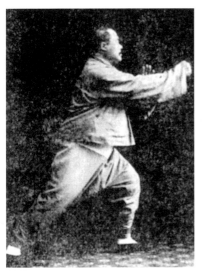

Section Fifty-One: Advance Step, Deflect, Parry, and Punch

The same as Section Sixteen.

Figure 51

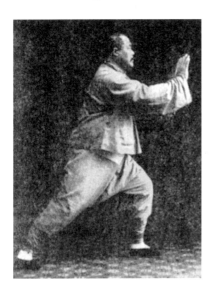

Section Fifty-Two: Like Sealing, As If Closing

The same as Section Seventeen.

Figure 52

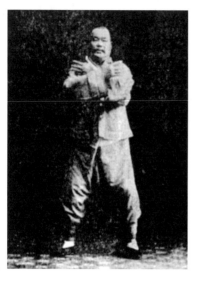

Figure 53

Section Fifty-Three: Cross Hands

This is the same as Section Eighteen.

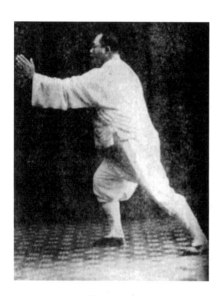

Figure 54

Section Fifty-Four: Embrace Tiger, Return to Mountain

This is the same as Section Nineteen.

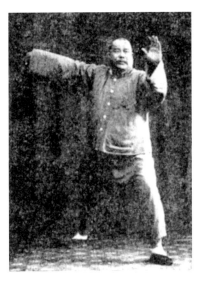

Figure 55

Section Fifty-Five: Oblique Single Whip

The Oblique Single Whip form is identical to the preceding Single Whip, except that the posture aligns obliquely with the corner direction. Therefore it is named Oblique Single Whip.

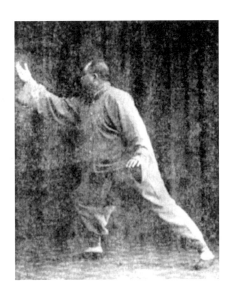

Figure 56

Section Fifty-Six: Wild Horse Parts Mane, Right Form

From the previous form, suppose an opponent comes from my right side and applies Push *(an)*. I then turn my body to the right, with my left foot also shifting in toward the right. The heel of the right foot simultaneously loosens, while the toes maintain an empty point of contact. Following, use the right hand to stick *(nian)* to the opponent's left and right wrists with a loosening motion slightly to the left side. Apply split *(lie)* to his right wrist with your left hand. At the same time, quickly advance the right foot, bending the knee and sitting solidly on it. The left leg extends straight. Follow by using the right forearm to separate out, striking below the opponent's armpit. In this way, his rooting strength *(gen li)* is pulled up *(ba qi)* by me, and then his body falls back! At this time, the left hand must also separate out to the rear, using sinking energy *(chenjin)* in order to balance the force of the right hand.

Translator's Comments

Note that the right arm draws downward to the left, offsetting the opponent's force from one's centerline, before opening and striking toward the right.

Section Fifty-Seven: Wild Horse Parts Mane, Left Form

The functions and purpose are the same as the right form with a change of direction.

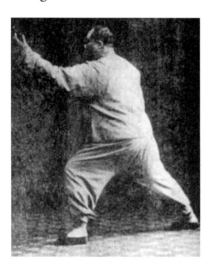

Translator's Comments

It is curious that there is no mention of a third Wild Horse Parts Mane form. In the received form, an odd number is prescribed, so that the transition to Grasp Sparrow's Tail proceeds from a Wild Horse Parts Mane, Right Form.

Figure 57

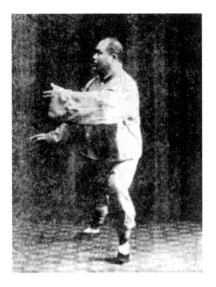

Figure 58

Section Fifty-Eight:
Grasp Sparrow's Tail
Same as preceding.

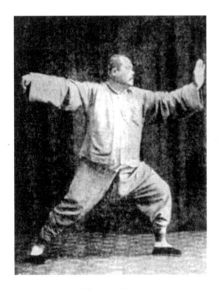

Figure 59

Section Fifty-Nine:
Single Whip
Same as preceding.

Section Sixty: Jade Maiden Threads Shuttle

From the Single Whip posture, suppose the opponent, from the right rear flank, uses his right hand to hit downward from above.

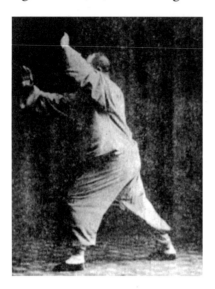

Figure 60

I then let my body follow the left foot in rotating together toward the right. The right foot subsequently lifts up and collects back, then lowers down in front of the left foot. The right foot separates out, the toes pointing to the right, and the weight settles into a full right stance. The left hand collects in, closing in under the right armpit. Following, it protectively encircles the right upper arm and threads past the right elbow. Then, using *pengjin,* the left arm turns toward the left front corner, engages the opponent's wrist, and wards it off upwardly *(pengqi).* The left leg concurrently advances, bends at the knee, and settles into a full left stance. The right foot extends straight. The right hand then changes into a palm, quickly threading forth beneath the left elbow, thrusting toward the opponent's rib cage and striking. There is no one who will not be dropped. In this form, the left and right hands thread reciprocally, suddenly hidden, suddenly appearing *(huyin huxian)* — unfathomable *(zhuo mo bu ding)* — attacking by seizing upon his emptiness. Thus, it is called Jade Maiden Threads Shuttle, in order to evoke the artfulness of the form.

Translator's Comments

The last few envoi statements, beginning with "There is no one who will not be dropped," do not appear in the earlier book, *Taijiquan shiyongfa,* and were evidently added by Zheng Manqing. The "suddenly hidden, suddenly appearing" (*huyin huxian* — 忽隱忽現) is a quote from the "Taijiquan Treatise."

Section Sixty-One: Jade Maiden Threads Shuttle, Two

Connecting with the previous form, if an opponent comes from my right rear to strike with his right hand directly at my head, I then

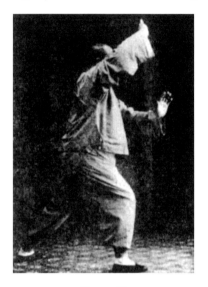

let my left foot turn inward somewhat. The right foot concurrently takes a step out to the right rear, with the leg bending at the knee, and becomes solid. The body accordingly pivots around (*ao zhuan)* to the right rear. The left leg changes to empty. Swiftly use the right wrist to stick fast to the outer edge of the opponent's right arm, and ward it off upwardly *(pengqi)* to the right. Following, bring the left hand to Push (*an)* toward the opponent's rib cage. The remaining aspects are the same as the preceding form.

Figure 61

Translator's Comments

The first Jade Maiden is toward the southwest. The second one is toward the southeast, so it involves a 270° clockwise turn.

Section Sixty-Two: Jade Maiden Threads Shuttle, Three

Connecting with the previous form, if an opponent comes from my left flank to strike with his left hand, I then let the toes of my right foot move out (*fen kai)* slightly to the right, sitting solidly.

The left foot lifts toward the left corner direction to step out, sitting solidly. The hand methods are the same as for the first form.

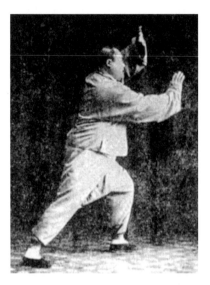

Figure 62

Translator's Comments

The third Jade Maiden proceeds with a 90° counter-clockwise turn to the northeast.

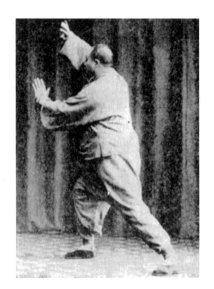

Figure 63

Section Sixty-Three: Jade Maiden Threads Shuttle, Four

This form is the same as the pre-ceding second form, except for the direction in which the Jade Maiden threads her shuttle. The formal postures *(zheng shi)* are to the four corners. There must be no mistake about this.

Translator's Comments

The final Jade Maiden is another 270° clock-wise turn, ending to face the northwest.

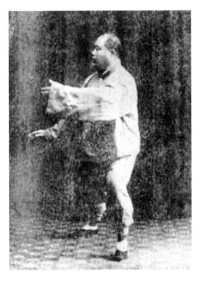

Figure 64

Section Sixty-Four:
Grasp Sparrow's Tail

As above.

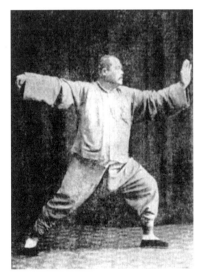

Figure 65

Section Sixty-Five:
Single Whip

As in Section Six, above.

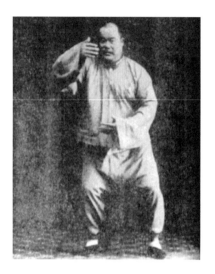

Section Sixty-Six:
Cloud Hands

The explanation and applications are as above.

Figure 66

Section Sixty-Seven: Single Whip, Squatting Single Whip

Single Whip is as above. From the point in Single Whip when one has already extended the left hand, if the opponent uses his right hand to push my left hand to the outside, or uses strength to grasp

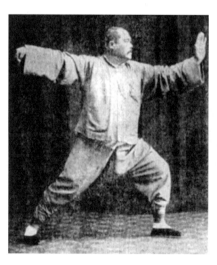

Figure 67a

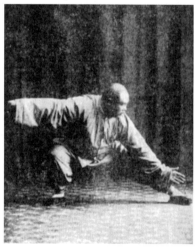

Figure 67b

firmly, I then let my right leg separate and open somewhat to the right. Sitting down toward the rear, my left hand simultaneously collects back to a point in front of my chest using round and lively *jin*. Perhaps the opponent uses his left hand to strike me. I then use my left hand to control his left wrist. I can either move it to the left or apply *cai* in a downward direction; both are possible. The right leg works simultaneously with the waist and *kua* in sitting down, in order to lead the other's strength while reserving my *qi*.

Translator's Comments

The instruction to let the leg separate and open refers to an initial turning out of the right foot and an opening of the stance in preparation for the sinking of the body into the low posture. The unified movement enables one to lead the opponent's strength (*qian bi zhi li* 牽彼之力), and reserve *xu* 蓄 one's *qi* 氣. The word *xu* means "to collect" or "to store," and it is the concept found in the "Mental Elucidation of the Thirteen Postures" in the line "Store energy (*xu jin* 蓄勁) as though drawing a bow."

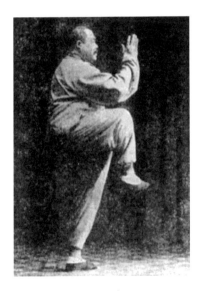

Figure 68

Section Sixty-Eight: Golden Cock Stands on One Leg, Right Form

From the preceding form, if the opponent hauls back with strength, I then take advantage of this *(shunshi)*, gathering my body forward and upward. My right leg accords with this movement, lifting upward, applying the toes of the foot to kick toward the opponent's abdomen. The right hand follows in advancing forward, bending at the elbow, with the fingers pointing upward. In this way, I close off the opponent's left hand. At this time, the left foot has become full, standing steady, while the right hand accords and advances. One can contain *(qianzhi)* the opponent's left or right hand. It is not necessary to hold or to grasp.

Translator's Comments

The phrase *shunshi* 順勢 can mean "to follow along with the force," or "to take advantage" of a situation. Both meanings apply here, but the context makes the latter rendering appropriate. One is virtually getting a free ride from the opponent.

The verb *qianzhi* 牽制, for the action taken with the right hand, means "contain, check, or restrain." It implies a light touch rather than a strong-arm tactic.

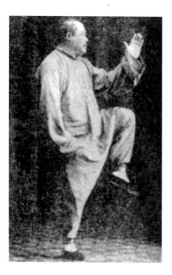

Figure 69

Section Sixty-Nine: Golden Cock Stands on One Leg, Left Form

From the right form, suppose the opponent uses his right fist to strike me. My right hand sinks down. Swiftly raise the left hand and lift *(tuo)* the opponent's elbow. Raise the left leg. It is the same as the right form.

Translator's Comments

The verb *tuo* 托 refers to using the heel of the palm to lift or hold something. Fu Zhongwen notes that this may be done as a martial application of the posture, but that in solo form training the fingers of the hand point up. (See my translation, *Fu Zhongwen: Mastering Yang Style Taijiquan,* pp. 141–142.)

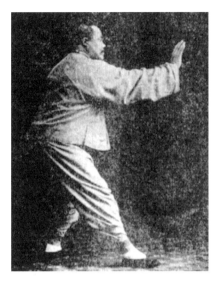

Section Seventy:
Step Back, Dispatch Monkey

The movements are identical with Sections Twenty-One and Twenty-Two above.

Figure 70

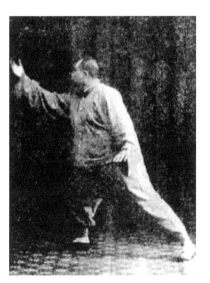

Section Seventy-One:
Flying Obliquely

Applications are the same as Section Twenty-Three above.

Figure 71

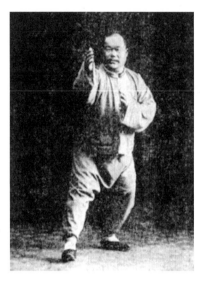

Figure 72

Section Seventy-Two:
Raise Hands Upward
The same as the above Section Seven.

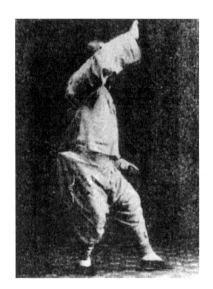

Figure 73

Section Seventy-Three:
White Crane Displays Wings
Same as above Section Eight.

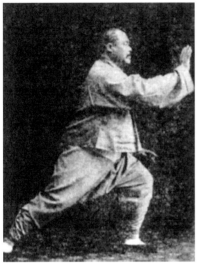

Figure 74

Section Seventy-Four: Brush Knee Twist Step

Same as above Section Nine.

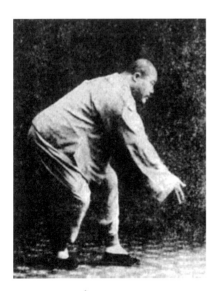

Figure 75

Section Seventy-Five: Needle at Sea Bottom

Same as above Section Twenty-Seven.

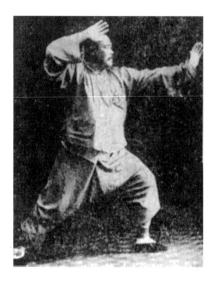

Section Seventy-Six: Fan Through Back

Same as above Section Twenty-Eight.

Figure 76

Section Seventy-Seven: Turn Body, White Snake Darts its Tongue

This form is somewhat similar to Turn Body and Strike, only the second form changes to a right palm application. One needs only to add sinking energy *(chenjin)* to the palm.

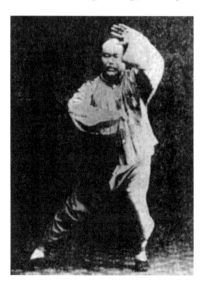

Figure 77a

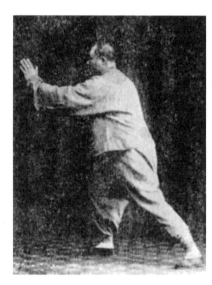

Figure 77b

Translator's Comments

Unfortunately, the photos do not clearly show the action of the right palm distinguishing White Snake Darts its Tongue from Turn Body and Strike (Section Twenty-Nine). In the received form the motion of the right arm is virtually the same, but instead of a back fist strike, the hand is held open.

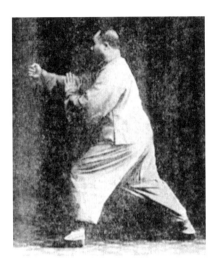

Figure 78

Section Seventy-Eight:
Deflect, Parry, and Punch

Same as above Section Thirty.

Section Seventy-Nine:
Grasp Sparrow's Tail

As above.

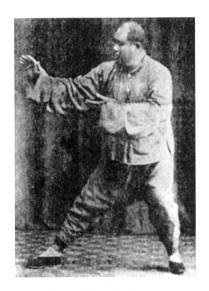

Figure 79

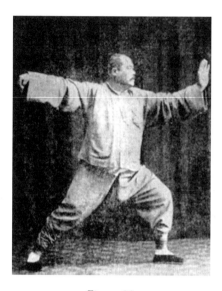

Figure 80

Section Eighty:
Single Whip
As above.

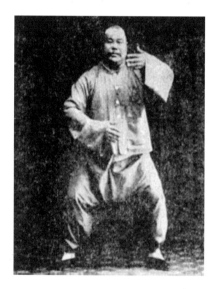

Figure 81

Section Eighty-One:
Cloud Hands
As above.

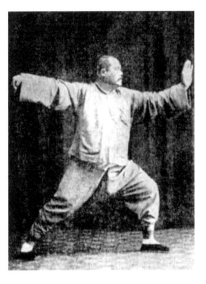

Section Eighty-Two: Single Whip

As above.

Figure 82

Section Eighty-Three: High Pat on Horse with Piercing Palm

The first part of the sequence is identical to Section Thirty-Five,

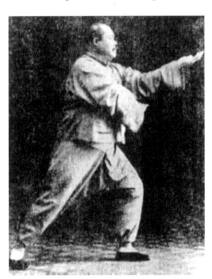

which may be consulted. However, after the right hand has probed forth *(tan chu)*, it then collects back, with the palm facing downward. The left hand lifts up slightly, and the piercing palm thrusts toward the opponent's throat. The right hand remains hidden beneath the left elbow, in order to respond to any changes *(yingbian)*.

Translator's Comments

Although the photo depicts the ending posture, the footwork

Figure 83

for the Piercing Palm is not described. The High Pat on Horse posture is rear-weighted—an empty left stance. The transition to the Piercing Palm requires stepping forward with the left foot and moving into a left bow stance. See *Fu Zhongwen: Mastering Yang Style Taijiquan*, pp. 146–147 for a detailed description.

Section Eighty-Four: Cross Legs

From the previous form, suppose the opponent uses his right hand to pull my right hand. I then draw my right hand clear until it

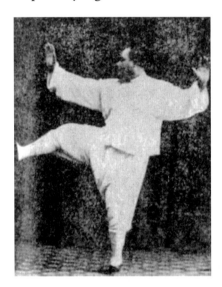

arrives beneath the left arm-pit. Following, I thrust my left palm toward the opponent's chest. Form Cross Hands. At this time, suppose there is an opponent at the right rear of my body, using his right hand to strike horizontally at me. I then swiftly turn my body around directly to the right. My left arm simultaneously turns over, bending at the elbow, as it forms an embrace with the right arm. I then swiftly separate and open my left and right hands to the front and rear, parrying *(lan zhu)* the opponent's hand. At the same time, swiftly raise the right leg upward. Use the heel of the foot to thrust *(deng)* toward the opponent's right flank. Then the opponent will surely react to my leg and will be sent bounding *(yue)* away!

Figure 84

Translator's Comments

The application scenario described involves two attackers. The drawing back of the right hand, combined with the rightward pivot of the body, pulls the first opponent to one's right and into one's left palm strike as though with centripetal force. The kick takes care of the second opponent. As with Section Thirty-Eight's Turn Body and Kick with Heel, the narrative here uses the phrase *ying tui* 應腿 with some productive ambiguity. Is this a "response/reaction" (*ying* 應) to the kicking leg, or is it a "response/reaction" within the attacker's legs as he bounds away, trying to regain equilibrium? The verb *yue* 躍 describes a spring-ing, leaping motion, familiar to those taijiquan practitioners who have been launched by a skilled opponent.

Section Eighty-Five: Advance Step, Punch Toward Groin

Connecting with the previous form, if the opponent, engaging in some back and forth, then withdraws his hand, I then lower my

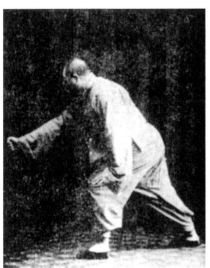

right foot. At the same time, the left foot advances forward, bending at the knee and sit-ting solidly. At this point, suppose the opponent comes again, kicking from below with his right foot. I quickly use my left hand to brush his foot to the outside of my left knee. My right hand there-upon forms a fist, which I direct toward the crotch of the opponent. The torso leans slightly forward.

Figure 85

Translator's Comments

This posture resembles Section Forty-One's Advance Step, Plant Punch, but the punch is not aimed as low in this case.

91

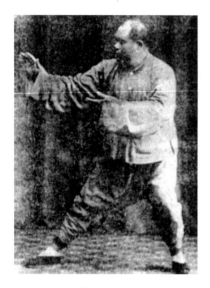

Section Eighty-Six: Advance Step, Grasp Sparrow's Tail

As above.

Figure 86

Section Eighty-Seven: Single Whip, Squatting Single Whip

As in Section Sixty-Seven.

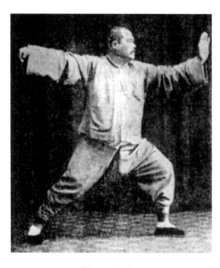

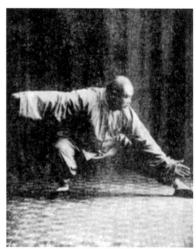

Figure 87a   Figure 87b

Section Eighty-Eight: Step Up to Seven Stars

From the previous form, suppose the opponent uses his right hand to chop downward from above. I then advance my body to the left and forward. The two hands change to fists and simultane-

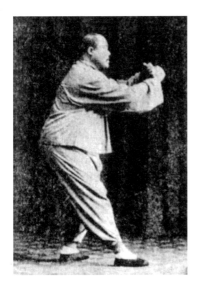

ously gather to intersect, forming the shape of the character seven (*qi* 七). With the hearts of the palms facing outward (to the sides), the arms ward off *(peng zhu).* One can also apply the fists in a direct strike to the opponent's chest.

Translator's Comments

Depending on the circumstance, this form can simply deflect an incoming fist, or it can advance to strike the solar plexus of the aggressor. It is a variation of the fundamental Cross-Hands form, but using fists instead of palms,

Figure 88

and with the ulna of the left wrist joining the radius of the right fist. In an early document said to have been transmitted by Yang Banhou, and translated by Douglas Wile as "Secrets of T'ai Chi Form Applications," it is said that this posture "forms a rack with the hands" (*jia shou* 架手). See Douglas Wile, *T'ai-chi Touchstones: Yang Family Secret Transmissions,* p. 61.

Section Eighty-Nine: Retreat Astride Tiger

From the previous form, suppose the opponent comes at me apply-ing *an* with both hands. I then allow my two wrists to adhere *(nian)* to the insides of the opponent's two wrists. My left hand splits open *(lie kai)* to the left downward direction. The right

93

hand sticks and lifts to the right upward direction. The two palms accordingly turn to face outward. The right foot follows with these

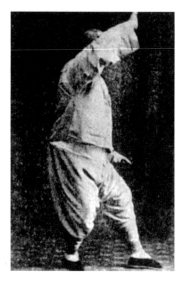

movements, retreating back a step, lowering down, and sitting solidly. The waist follows by sinking the *jin* downward. The left foot follows this by lifting upward, the toes touching the ground. This produces the Astride Tiger form, causing the entirety of the opponent's bodily strength to fall on emptiness. Now, although the opponent may be as fierce as a tiger, with but the slightest turning motion, he will be under my control.

Figure 89

Translator's Comments

The last two sentences—the envoi statement of the passage—do not appear in Yang Chengfu's earlier book, *Taijiquan shiyongfa,* but otherwise the description follows the original. Zheng Manqing may have added these remarks, but they differ slightly from the wording in own his book, *Taijiquan shisan pian* (Thirteen Chapters on Taijiquan), so one cannot be certain whether or not Yang was the source of the intriguing phrases "with but the slightest turning motion, he will be under my control." Again, the wording is consistent with what I have characterized "demonstration narrative" so could well have originated with Yang Chengfu.

Yang Zhenji observes in his book that the example photos used in his father's book for both Retreat Astride Tiger and White Crane Displays Wings are the same. He writes that the forms as transmitted are slightly different. In Zhenji's descriptions, White Crane Displays Wings shows the right hand closer to the temple, with the palm turned obliquely upward. In Retreat Astride Tiger, the right arm is a bit lower than the temple, and both arms are a bit more spread apart, left to right. It would seem that the photo here is the correct one for Retreat Astride Tiger. The outward spreading of the arms also serves as part of the set-up for the spin of Turn Body, Sweep Lotus, which follows.

Section Ninety: Turn Body, Sweep Lotus

From the previous form, suppose there is yet another opponent who is striking at me from the rear with a right fist. Respond-

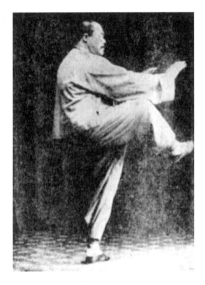

ing to opponents from both the front and rear, I am in a most urgent situation. So, I settle on my right foot. Then, lifting and suspending the left foot, I follow the rotation of my body to the right rear. At the same time, use the two hands with the left foot to employ whirlwind force *(xuan-feng shi)*. Apply the hands and foot to scrape *(gua)* the upper and lower areas of the rear oppo-nent. Upon returning in the turn to the original position, quickly adhere *(nian)* to the opponent's left elbow and wrist; follow and surround the opponent's wrist. Use roll back *(lu)* to lead to the left, split *(lie)* to pull back. Quickly, with the back of the right foot, kick the opponent's ribs, using transverse energy *(heng jin)*. The leg's movement is like a swift wind sweeping and rippling lotus leaves. What is called "soft waist" is as though it is absolutely without bone, loosened/relaxed *(sa)*, so that the entire body is the hands. The secret of this skill *(gong)* won't be understood by those who engage in superficial study.

Figure 90

Translator's Comments

The verb translated here as "rotation" is *xuanzhuan* 旋轉, which connotes spinning on an axis. The term "whirlwind force," *xuan-feng shi* 旋風勢, provides a vivid image of pivoting swiftly.

The last few sentences, beginning with the rather poetic simile "like a swift wind sweeping and rippling lotus leaves," are not present in Yang's earlier book and may have been added by Zheng Manqing. Zheng later wrote a poem titled "Song of Substance and Function" (Lo and Inn, trans., *Cheng Tzu's Thirteen Treatises on T'ai Chi Ch'uan*, pp. 217–218) in which we find the line "The whole body is a hand" (*hun shen shi shou* 渾身是手). There is also a line in Li Yiyu's "Ode to Sparring" on pp. 57, 133–134 of Wile's *Lost T'ai-chi Classics:* "My entire body is hands" (*man shen dou shi shou* 滿身都是手). These are the exact words used in the last half of the "boneless waist" sentence here in the Lotus Sweep section. A possible source for these words is a poem by Tang Shunzhi (1507–1560), a Neo-Confucian scholar-official, famous for fighting Japanese pirates along China's coast. Two lines in the poem read as follows:

百折連腰盡無骨，一撒通身皆是手。

With a hundred bends, even his waist seems completely boneless,
A loosening pervades his body, so that all of it is hand.

A translation of the Tang Shunzhi poem can be found in Wile's *T'ai Chi's Ancestors* (p. 13).

Section Ninety-One: Draw the Bow and Shoot the Tiger

From the previous form, suppose there is an instance of the opponent engaging in some back and forth, and withdrawing his body. I then allow my left and right hands to follow the opponent's hands, sticking fast, replying to and coiling around *(raoguo)* the opponent's wrists, whirling *(xuanzhuan)* them toward the right side. Form fists from the left corner and strike forth. The left hand, while sinking on the opponent's elbow (or forearm), strikes forth. The right leg accordingly lowers down, sitting solidly. The right hand

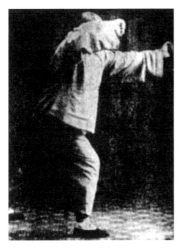

then strikes toward the opponent's chest. All of the above movements require reserving of one's power *(xu qi shi)* and the sinking of *jin* in the waist. It rather resembles a horse-riding posture. The left foot becomes empty. It is like forming a posture for shooting a tiger with a drawn bow.

Translator's Comments

Given the turned-out orientation of the right fist, the analogy of the

Figure 91

posture to drawing a bow is somewhat flawed, but in other respects the opening through the back and chest, and the set-up of tension between the two arms, does resemble the drawing of a large powerful bow.

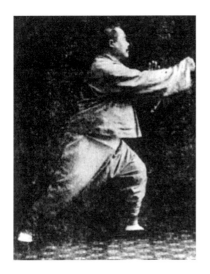

Section Ninety-Two: Advance Step, Deflect, Parry, and Punch

As above, Section Sixteen.

Figure 92

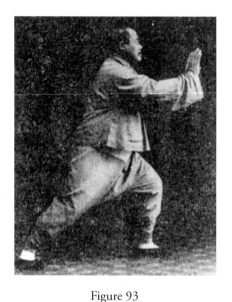

Section Ninety-Three:
Like Sealing, As If Closing

As above, Section Seventeen.

Figure 93

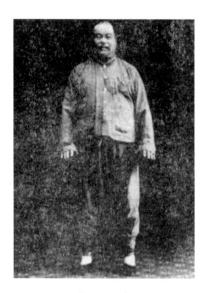

Figure 94

Section Ninety-Four:
Closing Form

From Like Sealing, As If Closing, change to Cross Hands. The two hands separate left and right and fall downward. The hearts of the palms face down as in the Beginning Form. This is named Closing Taiji. This is done when a complete *quan* set is finished.

Students must not overlook the fact that Closing Taiji means the uniting of Yin and Yang *(liang yi),* the four images *(si xiang)*, the eight trigrams *(ba gua)*, and the sixty-four hexagrams *(liu shi si gua)*, then again returning to Taiji. Also, it means collecting the mind and consciousness, the *qi* and the breath, to become whole and return to the *dantian*. Concentrate the spirit and still anxieties *(ning shen jing lu)*. Knowing when to stop with certainty *(zhi zhi you ding)*, you must not become scattered and lost, thus you will avoid making a fool of yourself before adepts.

Translator's Comments

In the above section, all of the wording following the basic description of the posture appears to have been added by Zheng Manqing. The fact that much of the added wording survives in the closing posture's description in Zheng's own later book, *Taijiquan shisan pian* (Thirteen Chapters on Taijiquan), gives weight to the theory that the additions were his.

Zheng may have felt a need to solemnify the closing posture. He achieved this by assembling a remarkable cluster of philosophical allusions. Collectively, the allusions serve as a sort of "amen" (in the sense of a formal affirmation) to the interior practice of the form.

The first allusion is to the cosmological imagery of the *Book of Changes,* specifically to a passage in the *Xicizhuan* (Appended Phrases), which may well be the *locus classicus* of the philosophical term "Taiji." The passage reads, "In Change there is the Supreme Polarity *(Taiji),* This gives rise to the Two Modes; the Two Modes give rise to the Four Images; the Four Images give rise to the Eight Trigrams." (Joseph A. Adler, trans., *Introduction to the Study of the Classic of Change,* by Chu Hsi, p. 15.) Zheng here paid tribute both to the name of the art and to the cosmological framework that has long enriched it.

Next, Zheng summons up important self-cultivation traditions by his use of the phrase *ningshen jinglu* 凝神静慮 ("concentrate the spirit and still anxieties"). One of the metaphorical models for consciousness in early Chinese texts is fluidity—the mind suffusing the body rather like a fluid. The concept of *qi* 氣 is often used in these contexts, with *qi* being a fluid-like conduit of consciousness. The fluid metaphor carries over into expressions such as one used for "concentration" — *ningshen*. *Ning* 凝 has fluid connotations of "coagulate," "condense," or "congeal." The term *ningshen* 凝神 appears in Chapter Nineteen of the *Zhuangzi*, in the sentence "He keeps his will undivided and concentrates his spirit." (Watson, *The Complete Works of Chuang Tzu*, p. 200.) Later, *ningshen* came to be used as a term for Daoist meditation. An early taiji text transmitted by Yang Banhou, *Quanti Dayong Jue* (The Greater Application of the Whole Body) — a formulaic inventory of the names and applications of the taijiquan postures — closes with some lines that highlight the internal requirements: "The greater application of the whole body is to make the intention primary (*quanti dayong yi wei zhu* 全體大用意為主). The body loosens, the *qi* is settled, and the spirit must concentrate" (*ti song qi gu shen yao ning* 體鬆氣固要神凝). (See Wile, *T'ai-chi Touchstones: Yang Family Secret Transmissions*, pp. 42–63, for a translation of the full text.)

Continuing with "knowing where to stop," Zheng makes a direct reference to a famous passage from the early Confucian text, the *Daxue*: "Knowing where to come to rest (*zhi zhi* 知止), one becomes steadfast (*you ding* 有定); being steadfast, one may find peace of mind; peace of mind may lead to serenity; this serenity makes reflection possible; only with reflection is one able to reach the resting place." (Daniel K. Gardner, trans., *Chu Hsi and the Ta-hsueh*, pp. 90–91.) The notion of "knowing where to stop" also appears in chapter 32 of the *Daodejing:* "By knowing when to stop you will avoid harm."

Finally, Zheng concludes with what at first seems a curious remark, that "you will avoid making a fool of yourself before adepts." This is an allusion to a story in the "Autumn Floods" chapter of the *Zhuangzi*. The chapter opens as the Lord of the Yellow River is about to meet Ruo, the God of the North Sea.

It is the time of the autumn floods, and the Lord of the River, fed by the hundred inland streams, is coursing eastward over the North China Plain. Brimming with self-satisfaction, and overcome with his own majesty and power, the Lord of the River suddenly reaches the North Sea. "Looking east, he could see no end to the water." Addressing Ruo, the God of the North Sea, he regrets his arrogance, and humbled by the "unfathomable vastness" of the ocean exclaims, "If I hadn't come to your gate, I would have been in danger. I would forever have been laughed at by the masters of the Great Method!" (Watson, *The Complete Works of Chuang Tzu,* p. 173.) Zheng Manqing's allusion to this story is especially interesting in light of the classical admonition that in taijiquan one should "move like a flowing river." Perhaps Zheng was suggesting that, while the student should indeed move like a flowing river, he or she should do so with a clear understanding of the tributary status of a river. One returns from motion to stillness, from the differentiated to the undifferentiated.

Push Hands and *Dalu* Sections

Push Hands

One: *Peng* Form

Taijiquan uses the practice of push hands *(tuishou)* to convey the meaning of its applications. Studying push hands, then, is learning how to sense energy *(jue jin)*. Once one can sense energy, it will not be difficult to understand energy *(dong jin)!* Hence the saying in the central treatise [Wang Zongyue's "Taijiquan Lun"], "From understanding energy, one then advances to spiritual illumination *(shenming)*." These words are without question rooted in push hands.

The following are photos of the four forms: *peng, lu, ji,* and *an;* namely, stick *(nian)*, join *(lian)*, adhere *(tie)*, and follow *(sui)*.

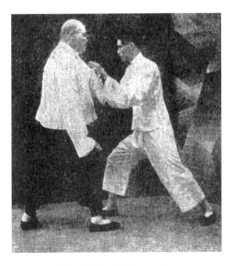

Push Hands Figure 1

These constitute the fixed-step push hands of yielding to another's initiative *(she ji cong ren)*. These pictures are of Zhaoqing [Yang Chengfu] and eldest son Zhenming [Yang Shouzhong] photographed together.

The method of *peng* (Ward Off) is facing outward, controlling and guarding against the push of the opponent, making it impossible for him to push as far as your chest or abdomen and adhere closely. Hence it is called *peng*. The meaning of this character *peng* is somewhat different from the definition in the *Shuowen*. *Peng* is a method, as in the picture. Left and right *peng* are identical in their application.

Avoid with the greatest caution being stiff and rigid. Also avoid being sluggish and heavy. Being stiff, one will not know one's own movement. Being sluggish, one will not know the opponent's intentions. Since one does not know one's self, one also does not know the other. This cannot be considered to be *tuishou!*

One who is sluggish and heavy necessarily uses strength to resist a person. This then becomes "dead hand" *(si shou)*. This is not what a taijiquan adept aspires to.

It must be said about *peng:* it is to adhere, not to resist *(kang)*. The hand *pengs* to the outside with the intent to adhere and answer. In addition, don't allow your *peng* hand to approach near the chest. Obtaining neutralizing energy *(hua jin)* relies entirely on the turning of the waist. Once I've turned my waist, my *peng* power *(peng shi)* is already complete!

Translator's Comments

The "definition in the *Shuowen*" alluded to above is perhaps the only known definition of the character *peng* 掤. Outside of taijiquan usage, the character *peng* is extremely rare. The *Shuowen Jiezi* is a famous etymological dictionary compiled circa 100 AD. The definition of *peng* in the *Shuowen* is " the cover of an arrow quiver," and the word appears in a poem in the *Shijing* (Book of Songs) with that meaning. (See Legge, trans., *The Chinese Classics,* Vol. IV, *The She King,* I:VII, pp. 129–131.) It is likely that the character was simply appropriated into taijiquan nomenclature as a term for the protective action of warding off. This same *Shuowen* definition had earlier been mentioned by Xu Yusheng, in the "Explanation of Names" section of his 1921 book, *Taijiquan shi tujie* (p. 52). Xu first defines the taijiquan term *peng* paronomastically, that is, by referring to a different word that is also pronounced *peng* 捧, and which may share some tangential meaning. Significantly, though, this *peng* means "to support" or "to receive respectfully with both hands" — an important gesture to understand for any exchange of money or gifts. Then, Xu's definition continues, "to bear upwardly" (上承), "to expand (膨 using another character pronounced *peng*) as though storing air in a leather ball." He then describes its function as leading the opponent's strength to fall into emptiness. Xu cites the entire *Shuowen* definition of *peng* as an arrow quiver cover, and a meaning of "using the hand to return an arrow," seeming to suggest some sort of correlation or analogous meaning in the taijiquan term. The author here, who was likely Zheng Manqing, is noncommittal on the relevance of the *Shuowen* definition

The remark about "dead hand" (*si shou* 死手) is a clever and dramatic contrast between genuine push hands and "dead hand," or lifeless technique resulting from the use of excess strength and resistance.

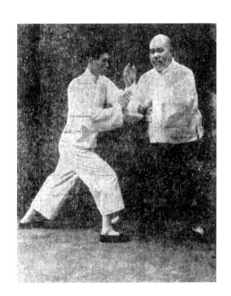

Push Hands Figure 2

Two: *Lu* Form

As for *lu* (Roll Back), I connect to my opponent's elbow with my wrist. Without resisting or pulling, I accord with the other's extended arm attacking me. I follow his force, and obtain it. This idea of push hands "collecting accounts" is what is called *lu*. This character also differs from the *Shuowen* dictionary; it is a specialized term of martial artists. The

105

method of *lu* is to turn the waist, adding a hand to connect to the area of the opponent's elbow, as in the above photo. One who is being rolled back must "give up the self and follow the other" *(she ji cong ren)*, yet must also know where to "give up the other and follow yourself" *(she ren cong ji)*. If the one being rolled back senses an increase of pressure from the opponent's hand, he can then take advantage and apply *kao* (Shoulder technique). Or if he senses a sudden break in the continuity of the other's Roll Back energy *(lujin)*, then he can swiftly let that side go, so that it is possible to attack using *ji* (Press).

Translator's Comments

The phrase *she ji cong ren* 舍己從人 has the meaning of "yield to the initiative of the other," but the more literal translation is "give up yourself and follow the other." The phrase is an important taijiquan aphorism appearing in the "Taijiquan Treatise," but it was actually borrowed from the *Mencius*, where it was used in more of a moral sense of accommodating the perspective of another person. (See Legge, trans., *The Chinese Classics*, Vol. II, *The Works of Mencius*, II A-8, p. 205.) The passage above is the only instance I've encountered where the phrase has been reversed to "give up the other and follow yourself" *(she ren cong ji* 舍人從己), which has a sort of tongue-in-cheek quality about it—a humorous way of making a point regarding the prerequisite of following the opponent's movements, but not to the extent of losing one's own equilibrium.

Three: *Ji* Form

As for *ji* (Press), it is precisely a counter to the Roll Back form. Roll Back thus lures this enemy's Push energy *(anjin)*, allowing him to enter my trap so that I get him. It's certain victory! But suppose the other first senses the force of my movement? The advancing *jin* of the opponent will surely stop mid-course, then change to a different posture. Now my Roll Back force has lost its effect. Therefore I must reverse my retreat to an advance, use the edge of

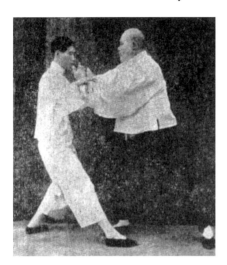

my forward arm to pluck *(cai)* his elbow. Raise the rearward hand and add it to the inside of the forearm, then seize the advantage and press forth *(ji chu)*. Now my opponent is caught in the midst of an abrupt change, and will most certainly lose his advantage as he receives my Press!

The one being pressed must remain calm *(zhending)* in the midst of the changes. If he is prescient *(you xianjue),* he will immediately void *(kong)* this Press energy *(jijin),* changing his posture to Push *(an)!*

Push Hands Figure 3

Translator's Comments

Note that, as with the narrative of the *lu* form, the form is explained from both the perspective of the partner performing the form and that of the opponent. As presented here, the techniques are less important than remaining calm (*zhending* 鎮定) in the midst of changes. The advice to be "prescient" (*xianjue* 先覺), that is, to anticipate and sense the opponent's changes in advance, is especially noteworthy. The emphasis is on sensing the opponent and being able to adapt to the circumstances.

Four: *An* Form

As for *an* (Push), since my Press posture didn't get an advantage, I then use my right hand so that it follows along the outer edge of my opponent's left arm and rolls onto his elbow.

Still producing a Roll Back form, I roll his arm back. If Roll Back again doesn't produce an advantage for me, then I turn over

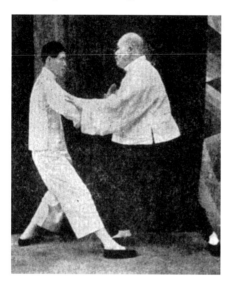

my right hand and use my palm to push on the opponent's left elbow joint, drawing it across. My left hand also pushes with the palm on his left wrist. This is what is called *an*.

With the completion of *an* one changes to perform *peng*. *Peng, lu, ji, an*—completing and then beginning again like a ceaselessly turning wheel. This is the idea of practicing stick *(nian)*, join

Push Hands Figure 4

(lian), adhere *(tie)*, and follow *(sui)*. The above four

postures have limitless transformations, and they are most difficult to describe in sufficient detail in writing. I hope that students will come to grasp the concepts through careful investigation. Along with the explanations given of the solo form skills, these particulars serve as insights to ease one's entry into this learning.

Translator's Comments

The closing remarks make it clear that, in the push hands context, the techniques of *peng, lu, ji,* and *an* should be understood as the syllabus in the course of study, while the more subtle level of skills—*nian, lian, tie,* and *sui*—constitute the learning objectives.

Illustrated Explanation of the *Dalu* Forms

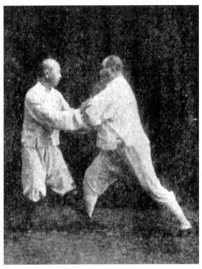

Peng Form

A is doing *peng.* **B** is doing *an.*

Dalu Figure 1

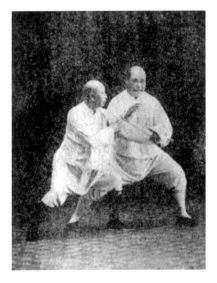

Lu Form

A's left hand does pluck *(cai),* while his right hand does compress *(jie).* Combining these forms makes the form *lie* (split). **B** is doing *kao* (Shoulder).

Dalu Figure 2

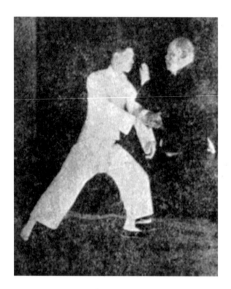

Cai Form

A's left-hand pluck is transitioning to *shan* (lightning strike). His right is still compressing *(qie jie)*. **B** uses his left elbow to fold *(zhe)*.

Dalu Figure 3

Ji Form

A Presses *(ji)*, then does Shoulder *(kao)*. The posture is the same as in Section Two

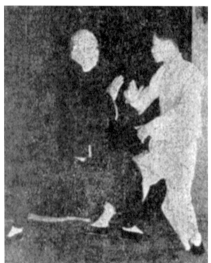

The four forms illustrated here mutually push and shift, in a continuously repeated process. The most important aspects of these forms are precisely in the nimble and subtle step changes. These free-flowing changes *(shen hua)*, however, can hardly be described in brush and ink. One must get the guidance of oral instructions, and then you will be able to plumb the transitions. Here, with refer-

Dalu Figure 4

ence to the illustrated explanations, the footwork and hand techniques are presented in the following.

Explanation of *Dalu* Four-Corner Push Hands

Four-corner push hands refers to the directions of *dalu,* with the shiftings and changes toward the four corners. It is different from the cardinal directionality of combined-step push hands. Combined-step push hands and *dalu,* taken together, are called "four-side, four-corner."

These correspond to the positions of the *bagua* (eight trigrams), named *Qian, Sun, Kan, Li,* and *Zhen, Dui, Gen, Kun.* In push hands, these are *peng, lu, ji, an, cai, lie, zhou,* and *kao.*

In the *dalu* starting form, the two partners stand opposite, facing either north-south or east-west, in a dual joined hand position. **A**, as in the first photo, is using *pengjin* (Ward Off energy) to neutralize *(hua)* **B**'s *anjin* (Push energy). Yielding at his left elbow and turning over his left wrist, he grasps **B**'s left wrist. This is *cai* (pluck). The right hand's position does not move, and then the hand compresses (*qie jie,* lit., to "cut off, interrupt"). A change then makes this into *lie* (split). *Lie* is to draw aside *(pie kai)* **B**'s left elbow and strike obliquely with the [left] palm toward the base of **B**'s neck. In regard to footwork, **A**'s front foot changes from full, as in Figure 1, to become empty. Advancing forward a bit, what was the rear foot becomes full and the other becomes empty, as in Figure 2. Here we have the change in application to *lu* (Roll Back). **A** performs *cai* (pluck). **B** does *kao* (Shoulder), as in Figure 2. Coming to Figure 3, this depicts the *cai* and *shan* forms. **A** releases the *caijin* in his left hand, then transforms it to *shan* (lightning strike). *Shan* is to aim the palm toward **B**'s face, prepared to strike. There is yet no movement in the footwork, as in Figure 3. Later, **B** lifts his left hand, withdrawing his left foot to align with his right foot. Swiftly, he again retreats back a step toward the left corner with the left foot, turning the torso so that the rear foot is sitting full.

Again, using his right hand, he rolls back **A**'s left hand. While **B**'s left hand plucks **A**'s left hand, **A** follows **B**'s retreating step. **A** then pursues with a step, lifting the left rear foot to temporarily align with the forward foot. Now it is time for **B** to again advance the next step. **A** quickly shifts his right foot to step toward the right front corner. Then he swiftly takes his left foot and inserts it below **B**'s crotch. Next, he adds his left shoulder to stick closely to **B**'s right arm, applying *kao*. This is advancing three steps, retreating two steps. In the middle, there is one step requiring the two feet to align side-by-side, then there is a change step to close up space, becoming the fourth section, as in Figure 4. The postures in Figure 4 and Figure 2 are the same. **A** and **B** each attack and defend in a round of changes, repeatedly turning, continuing to push, but with a changing step as in Figure 3, so that there is no redundancy. The four corners proceed in sequence. These are the *cai, lie, zhou,* and *kao* of *dalu.* These four hand methods have already been provided. However, among these four hand methods, there is none without application. All of these hand methods can issue *(fajin)*.

I hope that students will study carefully, according to the illustrations, so that they will reach understanding on their own.

Translator's Comments

Neither the Push Hands section nor the *Dalu* section should be construed as anything approaching a detailed description of the sequence or choreography of the forms. If the "nimble and subtle step changes" are key to understanding the *dalu* forms, the footwork is far from clear in this presentation. What is clear is that the author intended to present in broad strokes some of the basic potentialities within the changing forms, to point to connections with the solo form applications already suggested, and to urge the student to seek personal instruction and investigate the art through practice.

Appendix

I. The Taijiquan Treatise

Taiji, being born of *Wuji,* is the mother of *yin* and *yang.* In movement it differentiates; in stillness it consolidates. It is without excess or insufficiency. Follow, bend, then extend. When the other is hard, and I am soft, this is called yielding. I go along with the other. This is called adhering. To quick movements, I respond quickly. To slow movements, I follow slowly. Although the transformations have innumerable strands, this principle makes them as one thread. From careful investigation and experience, one may gradually realize how to comprehend energy *(dong jin).* From comprehending energy, you will attain by degrees spiritual illumination *(shen ming).* Nevertheless, without an exertion of effort over time *(yong li zhi jiu),* one will not be able to suddenly have a thorough understanding of it.

An intangible and lively energy lifts the crown of the head *(xu ling ding jin).* The *qi* sinks to the *dantian.* No leaning, no inclining. Suddenly hidden, suddenly appearing. When the left feels weight, then the left empties. When the right feels weight, then the right is gone. Looking up, it then becomes yet higher. Looking down, it then becomes yet deeper. Advancing, there is an even longer distance. Retreating, it is then even more crowded. One feather cannot be added. A fly cannot land. The other does not know me; I alone know the other. This is to be a hero with no adversaries along the way. Does it not all come from this?

There are many other kinds of martial arts. Although their forms are distinct from one another, overall they are nothing more than the strong taking advantage of the weak, or merely the slow yielding to the quick. Having strength to strike those without strength, the slow of hand giving way to the quick of hand—these are all from inherent natural ability, and bear no relationship to the capability that comes from earnest study. Examine the expression "Four ounces deflect one thousand pounds." Clearly this is not accomplished by means of strength. Observe a situation in which one who is aged can skillfully fend off *(yu)* a throng. How can this ability be one of speed?

Stand like a balance scale; active, like the wheel of a cart. Sink to one side, then follow. If double-weighted *(shuang zhong)*, then one will stagnate. Whenever we see those who for several years have perfected their skill, yet are unable to employ this neutralization and are generally overpowered by others, this is merely from not having come to understand the fault of double-weighting. If you want to avoid this fault, you must know *yin* and *yang*. To adhere is to yield; to yield is to adhere. *Yang* does not leave *yin; yin* does not leave *yang*. The mutual cooperation of *yin* and *yang* is precisely what makes up the understanding of energy *(dong jin)*. After comprehending energy, the more the practice, the greater the refinement. Silently memorize *(mo shi)* and ponder *(chuai mo)*, and gradually you will attain what you wish from your heart and mind *(cong xin suo yu)*. The foundation is to yield to the initiative of the other *(she ji cong ren)*. Many mistakenly forsake the near in pursuit of what is far away. It is said: "To be off in one's aim by the slightest fraction, one will lose the target by a thousand miles." The student must therefore be carefully discerning of the details herein. This comprises the treatise.

II. Song of the Thirteen Postures

The thirteen principal postures are not to be underestimated. The source of meaning is in the region of the waist.

You must pay attention to the turning transformations of empty and full, and the *qi* moving throughout your body without the slightest hindrance.

In the midst of stillness one comes in contact with movement, moving as though remaining still. According with one's opponent, the transformations appear wondrous.

For each and every posture, concentrate your mind and consider the meaning of the applications.

You will not get it without consciously expending a great deal of time and effort *(gongfu)*.

Moment by moment, keep the mind/heart *(xin)* on the waist. With the lower abdomen completely loosened, the *qi* will ascend on its own.

The coccyx *(wei lu)* is centrally aligned, and the spirit *(shen)* threads to the crown of the head. The whole body is light and nimble when the head is suspended at the crown.

Carefully concentrate upon your study. The bending, extending, opening and closing: let them come on their own.

Entering the gate and being led to the path, this must come from oral guidance. To ceaselessly exert oneself *(gongfu wu xi)* in the method is self-cultivation *(zi xiu)*.

If you ask, what are the criteria of essence and application? Intention *(yi)* and *qi* are the authority, bones and tissues the subjects.

If you want to find out where, in the end, the purpose lies, it is to increase longevity and extend one's years *(yi shou yan nian)*, a springtime of youth.

This song, oh, this song, has one hundred forty words. Every word is true and concise, there are no omissions.

If inquiry proceeds without regard to this, one's efforts *(gongfu)* will be wasted, and this will only cause one to sigh with regret.

III. The Mental Elucidation of the Thirteen Postures

Use the mind/heart *(xin)* to move the *qi*. You must cause it to sink soundly, then it can gather into the bones. Use the *qi* to move the body. You must cause it to accord smoothly, then it can easily follow your mind/heart *(xin)*. If the spirit of vitality *(jing shen)* can be raised, then there will be no apprehension of dullness or heaviness. This is what is meant by suspending the crown of the head. The intent *(yi)* and the *qi* must exchange with skillful sensitivity, then you will have a sense of roundness and liveliness. This is what is called the change of insubstantial and substantial. When issuing energy *(fa jin)*, one must sink soundly, loosen completely, and focus in one direction. In standing, the body must be centrally aligned, calm and at ease, supporting the eight directions. Move the *qi* as though through a pearl carved with a zigzag path (*jiu qu zhu,* literally, "nine-bend pearl"), reaching everywhere without a hitch. Mobilize *jin* (energy) that is like well-tempered steel, capable of breaking through any stronghold. One's form is like a hawk seizing a rabbit. One's spirit is like a cat seizing a rat. Be still like a mountain, move like a flowing river. Store energy *(xu jin)* as though drawing a bow. Issue energy *(fa jin)* as though releasing an arrow. Seek the straight in the curved. Store up, then issue. The strength issues from the spine; the steps follow the body's changes. To gather in is in fact to release. To break off is to again connect. In going to and fro there must be folding; in advancing and retreating there must be turning transitions. Arriving at the extreme of yielding softness, one afterward arrives at the extreme of solid hardness. With the ability to inhale and exhale will follow the ability to be nimble and lively. When the *qi* is cultivated in a straightforward manner, there will be no harm. When the energy *(jin)* is stored up in the curves, there will be a surplus. The mind/heart *(xin)* is the commander, the *qi* is the signal flag, the waist is the directional banner. First seek to open and expand, afterwards seek to draw up and gather together, then you will approach refinement.

It is also said, if the other does not move, I do not move. If the other moves slightly, I move first. The energy *(jin)* seems loosened *(song)* yet not loosened; about to expand, but not yet expanding. The energy *(jin)* breaks off, yet the intent *(yi)* does not. It is also said, first in the mind/heart, then in the body. The abdomen is loosened *(song)* so that the *qi* gathers into the bones. The spirit is at ease, the body calm. Carve this, each moment, into your mind/heart; remember closely: when one part moves, there is no part that does not move. When one part is still, there is no part that is not still. Leading the movements to and fro, the *qi* adheres to the back, then collects into the spine. Within, consolidate the spirit of vitality. Without, express tranquillity and ease. Step like a cat walking. Mobilize energy *(jin)* as though drawing silk. Throughout the whole body, the intent *(yi)* is on the spirit of vitality *(jing shen)*, not on the *qi*. If it is on the *qi*, then there will be stagnation. One who has it on the *qi* will have no strength. One who does not have it on the *qi* will attain pure hardness. *Qi* is like the wheel of a cart; the waist is like the wheel's axle.

IV. The Taijiquan Classic

Once in motion, the entire body should be light and agile, and even more importantly, must be threaded together *(guan chuan)*. The *qi* should be roused and made vibrant. The spirit *(shen)* should be collected within. Do not allow there to be any protuberances or hollows. Do not allow there to be any intermittence. It is rooted in the feet, issued by the legs, governed by the waist, and expressed in the fingers. From the feet, to the legs, then to the waist, always there must be complete integration into one *qi*. In advancing forward and retreating back, you will then be able to seize the opportunity and the strategic advantage *(de ji de shi)*. In a case of not gaining the opportunity and strategic advantage, your body will become scattered and confused. The flaw in this case must certainly be sought in the waist and legs. This is so whether up or down, forward or backward, left or right. These cases are all of mind intent *(yi)* and do not refer to the external. When there is up, then there is down. When there is forward, then there is backward. When there is left, then there is right. If the intent is to go upward, then direct the mind intent downward, just as, if one is going to lift an object, then one in addition applies to it the force of a downward push. Thus, its root will be severed, and it will be collapsed quickly and decisively. Insubstantial and substantial must be clearly distinguished. Each point has its point of insubstantial/substantial. Everywhere there is always this one insubstantial/substantial. The entire body is threaded together joint by joint *(jie jie guan chuan)*. Do not allow the slightest interruption.

What is Long Boxing *(chang quan)?* It is like the Long River, or a great ocean, flowing smoothly and ceaselessly. Ward Off *(peng)*, Roll Back *(lu)*, Press *(ji)*, Push *(an)*, Pull Down *(cai)*; Rend *(lie)*, Elbow Stroke *(zhou)*, Shoulder Stroke *(kao)*: these are the Eight Trigrams *(ba gua)*. Advance, Retreat, Look Left, Gaze Right, Central Equilibrium: these are the Five Phases *(wu xing)*. *Peng, Lu, Ji,* and *An,* accordingly, are [the Trigrams] *Qian, Kun, Kan,* and *Li,* or the four cardinal directions. *Cai, Lie, Zhou,* and *Kao,* then, are [the Trigrams] *Sun, Zhen, Dui,* and *Ken,* or the four corner directions. Advance, Retreat, Look Left, Gaze Right, and Central Equilibrium, accordingly, are Metal, Wood, Water, Fire, and Earth. Taken together, these comprise the Thirteen Postures.

V. The Song of Pushing Hands

In Ward Off *(peng)*, Roll Back *(lu)*, Press *(ji)*, and Push *(an)*, you must be conscientious.

Upper and lower follow one another; the other has difficulty advancing.

Let him come and strike with great strength.

Lead his movement, using four ounces to deflect a thousand pounds.

Attract him into emptiness, join, then issue.

Adhere, connect, stick, follow, without letting go or resisting.

BIBLIOGRAPHY

Adler, Joseph A., trans., Chu Hsi, *Introduction to the Study of the Classic of Change (I-hsueh ch'i-meng)*. New York: Global Scholarly Publications, 2002.

Allan, Sarah. *The Way of Water and Sprouts of Virtue*. Albany: State University of New York Press, 1997.

Ames, Roger T., and Rosemont, Henry, Jr., trans. *The Analects of Confucius: A Philosophical Translation*. New York: Ballantine Books, 1998.

Ames, Roger T. *The Art of Rulership: A Study of Ancient Chinese Political Thought*. Albany: State University of New York Press, 1994.

Ames, Roger T., trans. *Sun-Tzu: The Art of Warfare*. New York: Ballantine Books, 1993.

Brownell, Susan. *Training the Body for China: Sports in the Moral Order of the People's Republic*. Chicago: University of Chicago Press, 1995.

Chan, Wing-tsit. *A Source Book in Chinese Philosophy*. Princeton: Princeton University Press, 1963.

Chang, Hao. *Liang Ch'i-ch'ao and Intellectual Transition in China, 1890–1907*. Cambridge: Harvard University Press, 1971.

Davis, Barbara. *The Taijiquan Classics: An Annotated Translation, Including a Commentary by Chen Weiming*. Berkeley: North Atlantic Books, 2004.

Fu Zhongwen. *Yang shi taijiquan* (Yang Style Taijiquan). Hong Kong: Xianggang Taiping Shuju, 1968. Originally published 1963.

Gardner, Daniel K. *Chu Hsi and the Ta-hsueh: Neo-Confucian Reflection on the Confucian Canon*. Cambridge: Harvard University Press, 1986.

Graham, A. C. *The Book of Lieh-tzu: A Classic of Tao*. New York: Columbia University Press Morningside Edition, 1960, 1990.

Hall, David L., and Ames, Roger T. *Anticipating China: Thinking Through the Narratives of Chinese and Western Culture.* Albany: State University of New York Press, 1995.

Hanyu da cidian (The Great Chinese Word Dictionary). Hong Kong: Shangwu/Commercial Press, CD-ROM version, 1998.

Huang Wen-Shan. *Fundamentals of T'ai Chi Ch'uan,* Third Edition. Hong Kong: South Sky Book Company, 1979.

Ishida Hidemi. "Body and Mind: The Chinese Perspective." In Livia Kohn, ed., *Taoist Meditation and Longevity Techniques.* Ann Arbor, MI: Michigan Monographs in Chinese Studies, 1989, pp. 41–71.

Jullien, Francois. *The Propensity of Things: Toward a History of Efficacy in China.* New York: Zone Books, 1995.

Knoblock, John. *Xunzi: A Translation and Study of the Complete Works, Volume I.* Stanford, CA: Stanford University Press, 1988.

Legge, James. *The Chinese Classics.* Hong Kong: Hong Kong University Press, 1861–73; Reprint, Taipei: Southern Materials Center, 1985.

_____. *Li Chi: Book of Rites.* New Hyde Park, NY: University Books (Reprint), 1967.

Lo, Benjamin Pang Jeng, and Inn, Martin, trans. *Cheng Tzu's Thirteen Treatises on T'ai Chi Ch'uan.* Berkeley, CA: North Atlantic Books, 1985.

Lynn, Richard John. *The Classic of Changes: A New Translation of the I Ching.* New York: Columbia University Press, 1994.

Oshima, Harold. "A Metaphorical Analysis of the Concept of Mind in the *Chuang-tzu.*" In Victor H. Mair, ed., *Experimental Essays on Chuang-tzu,* University of Hawaii Press, 1983, pp. 63–84.

Pang, T.Y. *On Tai Chi Chuan.* Bellingham, WA: Azalea Press, 1987.

Rutt, Richard. *Zhouyi: The Book of Changes.* London: Routledge Curzon, 2002.

Sawyer, Ralph D. *The Seven Military Classics of Ancient China, Including The Art of War.* Boulder, CO: Westview Press, 1993.

Schipper, Kristofer. *The Taoist Body,* trans. Karen C. Duval. Berkeley: University of California Press, 1993.

Selby, Stephen. *Chinese Archery.* Hong Kong: Hong Kong University Press, 2000.

She Gongbao. *Jingxuan taijiquan cidian* (Dictionary of Essential Taijiquan Terminology). Beijing: Renmin Tiyu Chubanshe, 1999.

Swaim, Louis, trans. *Fu Zhongwen: Mastering Yang Style Taijiquan.* Berkeley, CA: North Atlantic Books, 1999.

Watson, Burton. *The Complete Works of Chuang Tzu.* New York: Columbia University Press, 1968.

Watson, Burton. *Records of the Historian: Chapters from the Shih-chi of Ssu-ma Ch'ien.* New York: Columbia University Press, 1969.

Wile, Douglas. *Cheng Man-Ch'ing's Advanced T'ai-Chi Form Instructions.* Brooklyn: Sweet Ch'i Press, 1985.

_____. *Master Cheng's Thirteen Chapters on T'ai Chi Ch'uan.* Brooklyn: Sweet Ch'i Press, 1982.

_____. *Lost T'ai-chi Classics from the Late Ch'ing Dynasty.* Albany: State University of New York Press, 1996.

_____. *T'ai Chi's Ancestors: The Making of an Internal Martial Art.* Brooklyn: Sweet Ch'i Press, 1999.

_____, trans. *T'ai-chi Touchstones: Yang Family Secret Tranmissions,* revised ed. Brooklyn: Sweet Ch'i Press, 1983.

Wu Zhiqing. *Taiji zhengzong* (Orthodox Taiji). Shanghai: Shanghai Shuju Chubanshe, 1985. Originally published 1940.

Xu Longhou (Yusheng). *Taijiquan shi tujie* (Taijiquan Forms Illustrated). Taibei: Hualian Chubanshe, 1982. Originally published 1921.

Xu Shen. *Shuowen jiezi* (a comprehensive Han dynasty dictionary, c. 100 AD). Hong Kong: Zhonghua Shangwu Shuju, 1972.

Yang Chengfu. *Taijiquan shiyongfa* (Application Methods of Taijiquan). Reprinted as *Taijiquan Yongfa Tujie.* Taibei: Wuzhou Chubanshe, 1996. Originally published 1931.

_____ . *Taijiquan tiyong quanshu* (Complete Book of the Essence and Applications of Taijiquan). Hong Kong: Zhenshanmei Chubanshe, n.d., & newly typeset edition, Taibei: Wu Xue Shu Guan (Lion Books), 2001. Originally published 1934.

Yang Zhenduo. *Yang Style Taijiquan* (English Edition). Beijing: Morning Glory Publishers, 1996.

_____. *Zhongguo Yang shi taiji.* Xian: Shijie Tushu Chuban Gongsi, 1997.

Yang Zhenji. *Yang Chengfu shi taijiquan* (Yang Chengfu Style Taijiquan). Guangxi: Guangxi Minzu Chubanshe, 1993.

Zheng Manqing. *Zhengzi taijiquan shisan pian* (Master Zheng's Thirteen Chapters on Taijiquan). Taipei: Shizhong quan she, 1950.

About North Atlantic Books

North Atlantic Books (NAB) is a 501(c)(3) nonprofit publisher committed to a bold exploration of the relationships between mind, body, spirit, culture, and nature. Founded in 1974, NAB aims to nurture a holistic view of the arts, sciences, humanities, and healing. To make a donation or to learn more about our books, authors, events, and newsletter, please visit www.northatlanticbooks.com.